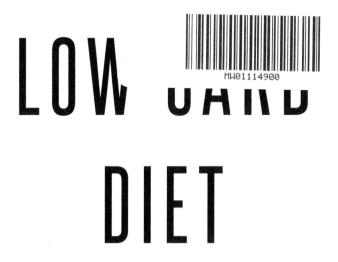

LOW CARB

DIET

- 3 Books in 1 -

Keto For Women Over 50.

Keto Diet After 50.

Keto Diet Cookboook After 50.

How to Reset Your Metabolism, Burn Fat, Lose Weight, Deflate the Belly, Get Body Confidence and Boost Your Energy After 50.

ALICE HARWING

TABLE OF CONTENTS

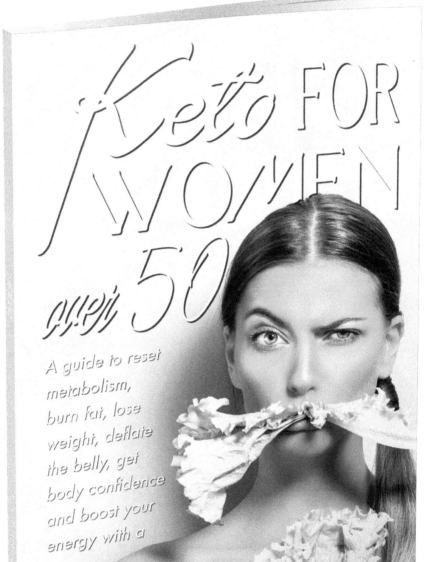

Keto FOR WOMEN over 50

A guide to reset metabolism, burn fat, lose weight, deflate the belly, get body confidence and boost your energy with a tasty meal plan

ALICE HARWING

KETO FOR WOMEN OVER 50

A guide to reset metabolism, burn fat, lose weight, prevent diabetes get body confidence and boost your energy with a tasty meal plan

ALICE HARWING

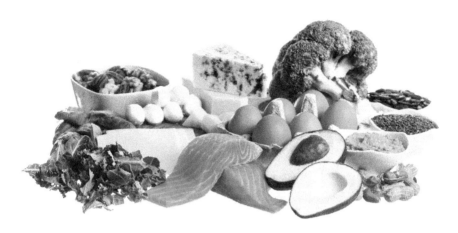

Introduction

The ketogenic diet is an "old-fashioned" diet developed as an alternative therapy for childhood epilepsy and can now be used to promote rapid weight loss, especially in severe obesity, and to treat various pathologies, including diabetes and neurodegenerative diseases. It was born almost 100 years ago and became popular in the 1920s and 1930s as an alternative to childhood epilepsy therapy. It was Dr. Russell Wilder of the Mayo Clinic who theorized about the properties of this diet in 1924 and published the first scientific data on his experiments.

In the 1940s, its use in the treatment of childhood epilepsy became obsolete due to the introduction of a new antiepileptic drug on the market. Harvard University Professor Blackburn's groundbreaking study in the 1970s began to spread and use the ketogenic diet protocol to treat obesity around the world.

Numerous studies have shown that the ketogenic diet can increase weight loss, improve health, and even have benefits in treating diabetes, epilepsy, and Alzheimer's. There is a variety of scientific evidence on the effectiveness of the ketogenic diet for losing weight, reducing body fat, and maintaining muscle mass.

Several studies have compared low-fat diets to ketogenic diets to assess weight loss performance, and the results show the superiority of the ketogenic diet. A 2013 randomized study published by JCEM identified the effects of a low-carbohydrate diet on body composition and cardiovascular risk factors in 42 overweight women. Women who follow the ketogenic diet have been found to lose 2.2 times more weight than low-calorie, low-fat women (equivalent to 30%). It also shows elevated levels of triglycerides and HDL (good) cholesterol.

The ketogenic diet can increase body weight loss, reduce excess fat, and increase insulin sensitivity. All of these are factors that are strongly associated with type 2 diabetes, prediabetic syndrome, and metabolic syndrome.

The diet offers tremendous benefits for a variety of neurodegenerative diseases, including Alzheimer's and Parkinson's disease, and may also offer protection against traumatic brain injuries and strokes.

This observation is supported by studies in animal models showing how the ketone body, especially β-hydroxybutyrate, offers nerve protection against various types of cell damage. The ketogenic diet is a dietary therapy for the treatment of epilepsy in children, and due to the reduction in insulin-related levels, it can also be an excellent strategy for polycystic ovaries and acne.

The ketogenic diet consists of a "total reorganization of the metabolism", and it is a process not without health risks: in one of the two studies, in fact, a greater propensity to obesity emerged in the mice fed the ketogenic diet. The difference with the positive effects manifested in the other case is due to the different choices that the researchers made during the experimentation phase: on the one hand, we opted to alternate the ketogenic diet and the usual diet, on the other, the caloric intake was limited to avoid weight gain.

The ketogenic diet would also improve long-term memory and longevity. For now, however, it has only been shown in mice. That ketogenic diets are now considered miracle weight loss is a fact, although we must always remember that for every diet we decide to follow, we must have a healthy dose of skepticism.

CHAPTER 01

WHAT IS KETOGENIC DIET AND HOW IT WORKS ?

Chapter01 - What Is Ketogenic Diet and how it Works?

A diet that results in the production of ketone bodies by the liver is known as a ketogenic diet; causes your system to use fat instead of carbohydrates for energy. Limit carbohydrate intake to a low level causing some reactions. However, it is not a high protein diet. It involves a moderate protein intake, low carbohydrate content, and high fat content. The exact percentage of macronutrients will vary based on your needs. Fat makes up 75 percent of the calories you eat; therefore, it is a fundamental component of the diet, proteins occupy 30% of the calories you eat and carbohydrates 10%.

Your system generally works on a mixture of protein, carbohydrates, and fat. This diet eliminates carbohydrates, which depletes your system reserves and the body finds an alternative source of energy. Many of your organs can use free fatty acids, but not all of them can use ketone bodies, for example, the brain and nervous system.

Insufficient free fatty acid disintegrations release ketone by-product bodies. The energy supplied is obtained from non-carbohydrate fats, which are used by organs such as the brain. As a consequence of the rapid manufacture of ketone bodies, which causes them to accumulate in the blood, ketosis develops. The manufacture and use of glucose in your system is reduced; the protein used to generate energy is also reduced.

Glucagon and glucose levels are affected by ketogenic diets. Insulin turns glucose into glycogen that is recycled as fat, while glucagon turns glycogen into glucose to provide energy for your system. Eliminating carbohydrates from the diet improves glucagon levels and lowers insulin levels. This, in the end, causes the release of a greater number of FFAs and their breakdown in the liver that results in the manufacture of ketone bodies and induces the state of ketosis.

The diet is, in a way, identical to starvation, with the distinction being that food eaten in one. The metabolic impacts that come about and the adjustments experienced in starvation are approximately the same as those experienced during the diet. There has been an extensive study of the reaction to complete hunger, probably more so than the diet on its own. That's why the vast bulk of the information described is derived from the analyses of fasting individuals. There are few exceptions, but the diet's metabolic impacts are similar to those that occur during starvation. The reactions in ketosis as a result of carb restriction are the same as the reactions seen with starvation. In this regard, protein and fat amounts are not that important.

Considering how carbs are not wanted in this diet, it may leave you wondering how much is needed for daily sustenance by your system. The body undergoes at least three significant adjustments when carbs are taken away from the diet to preserve the little glucose and protein it has. The principal adjustment is a general change in power source to FFA from glucose in most of your organs. This change spares the slight quantity of glucose accessible to power the brain. In the leukocytes, erythrocytes, and bone marrow that continue to use glucose, the second adaptation happens. These tissues break down glucose partly to lactate and pyruvate that go to the liver and are transferred back to glucose to avoid the depletion of accessible glucose reserve. Therefore, this issue doesn't end in a large decrease of glucose in your system and can be ignored in terms of the carbs need of the body. The third, and likely the most important, adjustment happens in your body, which, by the third week of continuous ketosis, transforms to the use of ketones for 75% of the power demands instead of getting from carbs. Since the brain continuously depletes glucose in the body, the regular carbohydrate demands are all that we need to bother ourselves with.

Your brain uses about 100 g of glucose daily in regular conditions. This implies that any diet that is based on fewer than 100 g of carbs daily will cause ketosis, the level of which depends on how many carbs are consumed that is the fewer carbs eaten, the greater the ketosis. Eating carbs below 100 grams will result in ketosis. With the continued adaptation of the brain to the use of ketones for power and the glucose demands of your system decline, fewer carbs should be absorbed to sustain the ketosis state.

There is no one-size-fits-all when it comes to how much of your total calorie requirement you should derive from carbs. Some nutritionists advise that people keep it in the low end, which is five percent, but it is not necessarily good advice as the exact amount depends on your system. To get the right amount for you will have to rely on the trial and error method. Select a percentage and see how it feels for you; if you don't like the results, you can adjust accordingly. With fats and protein, just like in carbs, there is no exact amount for everyone. It all depends on you, but seventy-five percent is a good place to start.

There is no space to' cheat' your diet here. You should follow it completely as even one meal that does not follow its rules can slow down your advancement for about a week as your body is withdrawn from ketosis. Always make sure you've eaten enough so that you will not be tempted to have a snack that could ruin all you've been working for.

Chapter 02-Understanding your Body

METABOLISM

As women age, their metabolism naturally slows down by approximately 50 calories per day. This means that you need to consume fewer calories if you maintain the same level of activity.

While 50 calories may not seem like a lot, think about how long it takes and the amount of effort required to burn the same amount. According to the National Institute of Health (NIH), to lose one pound of fat per week, an average person must create a 500 calorie per day deficit. In other words, burn more calories than you consume.

As your metabolism slows down, and as we've mentioned, it could slow by 50 calories per day, it would require a deficit of 550 calories per day (or 3,850 calories per week) to lose just one pound of fat. This sounds daunting, and for many, this fact alone will cause them to give up.

MUSCLE LOSS

As people age, it is natural for both women and men to lose lean muscle mass. This has the effect of slowing the metabolism as well as lessens strength and mobility. Although there is no way to stop the body from losing muscle, the progression can be slowed with exercise, specifically resistance and strength training.

Studies have shown that when you increase your muscle mass, you boost your resting metabolism at any age. In other words, you can burn more calories while resting simply by adding weight training to your workout regimen.

If you are a woman in your fifties and have never considered building those muscles, this may be a great time to start. However, it is highly advised that you consult with your doctor before adding resistance training to your workout.

MEN VERSUS WOMEN

While it may seem that men do not experience the same weight gain/loss struggles as women, they certainly do have their struggles.

A man's metabolism slows down as well as the ages. The difference is that men do not experience the same hormonal changes, which play a major role in metabolism, weight loss, and muscle degeneration.

During menopause, when estrogen levels decrease, fat storage is promoted around. While you may have struggled your entire life with weight gain in your hips and thighs, this new fat in your belly area is not only more difficult to lose but brings with it additional health risks to your heart and organs.

Body Aches

It is natural that as you age, you are less willing to engage in physical activity. While your brain may be telling you to exercise more frequently, your body may be sending you signals that it is not ready or capable of exercise.

It is not uncommon for women to have aches and pains in their 50s and beyond that were not there just a few short years ago. From inflamed knees to achy hips and sore muscles, these body aches may hinder your ability to get out there and move. However, it is important to note that while you may have these issues NOW, they will only get worse if you do not take the initiative to exercise and manage your weight.

With added weight comes added pressure on joints and bones, making them less resilient, more inflamed, and possibly even more painful. Take control of your body and your future now to avoid many of the weight induced complications that women may experience, including diabetes, high blood pressure, certain cancers, stroke, arthritis, and heart disease.

Mental Block

For some women, weight gain has never been an issue. With an active lifestyle and healthy eating, they have always been able to maintain a healthy weight appropriate for their body type.

Unfortunately, for them, the idea that the body has shifted out of their control is a mental challenge.

Everyone has that friend. She was super skinny in high school, shapely and athletic in college, even surprisingly bounced back after giving birth to her children. Suddenly her body has decided that it no longer can maintain that metabolism level, and now that she is in her fifties, she has no way of knowing how to manage her weight.

For her, it may be a mental challenge to now have to control this part of her body that always seemed just to function properly. She never had to put any thought or effort into her eating habits or exercise routine. The fact that she now has to be concerned causes a mental block making it more difficult to maintain control of her weight.

While you may have been envious of her before, age seems to have a leveling effect. We are all going to do it! There is no avoiding it, so why not take steps to take control of your weight, manage your health, and increase your longevity.

Unfortunately, calorie counting is difficult enough, but combining this with less exercise and the natural occurrence of muscular degeneration, you can see how women over 50 may struggle with weight loss!

The premise of this guidebook is to provide women over 50 with a healthy alternative way of eating to remain healthy and increase their chances of longevity. It also assumes that you do not suffer from health issues that may prohibit you from eating certain foods and from exercising.

BENEFITS OF KETO FOR WOMEN OVER 50

While the keto way of eating is beneficial for anyone at any age, for women of 50, it can have dramatic and even life-saving benefits.

•	Abdominal fat. Yes, I said it! There is no denying that as we age, we all tend to get a little more around the middle. Otherwise known as visceral fat, it is not only difficult to lose but increases the risk of health problems.

Keto increases fat burning, specifically targeting abdominal fat.

•	Insulin sensitivity. As you consume carbohydrates, they are naturally converted into glucose, which is then transported by insulin throughout the body. With age, the body's sensitivity to insulin decreases, increasing the risk of Type 2 diabetes.

Keto increases insulin sensitivity and thereby reduces the risk of developing diabetes.

•	Reduced inflammation. Inflammation is part of the body's natural healing process. As women age, it can occur more frequently, causing pain and discomfort.

Keto, as a high-fat diet, can have a dramatic impact on reducing inflammation.

•	Brain function. As the female body ages, reduced hormone levels can cause women to experience mood swings, memory loss, difficulty concentrating, and can even trigger depression and anxiety.

The Keto diet provides the brain with an alternate source of fuel in ketones.

- Improved cardiovascular health. Increased levels of triglycerides and "bad" cholesterol puts women over 50 at a higher risk of heart disease.

Keto is a low-carb diet that reduces triglycerides and increases "good" cholesterol, thereby reducing the risk of heart disease.

- Decreased blood pressure. Although it is common for women to have lower blood pressure levels than men, it does tend to increase with age. High blood pressure brings additional risks of heart disease, stroke, and even kidney disease.

Keto is a low-carb diet, can help to reduce blood pressure.

- Muscle loss. As women age, they naturally tend to lose muscle mass, which further reduces metabolism. Muscle loss can also prevent a woman from being physically active.

Keto provides a higher amount of protein, which is critical for muscle mass and to prevent loss.

- Increased bone density. Women are prone to lose bone mass, which can lead to osteoporosis, the key factor in bone weakness and fracture.

Keto can help improve bone strength and density with its high levels of calcium-rich leafy greens.

Keto diet is not only beneficial to women for weight loss. However, it has so many added benefits that not implementing keto as a lifestyle may be detrimental to the health of a woman over 50!

It is important to note that you should consult with your physician before starting a new diet and exercise regimen. Nothing contained in this guidebook should be considered medical advice, nor is it a guarantee that you will reap the benefits as described.

All of the recipes contained herein can be cooked in less than 30 minutes and are made with good, wholesome ingredients. Whether you are new to keto or have experience with keto, these recipes will surprise you. If you want to go keto, but do not know where to start, then this is your go-to guide. Start to lose weight and gain a healthy lifestyle today!

By considering keto to be a lifestyle, not a diet, you will be well on your way to weight loss and living a healthier lifestyle.

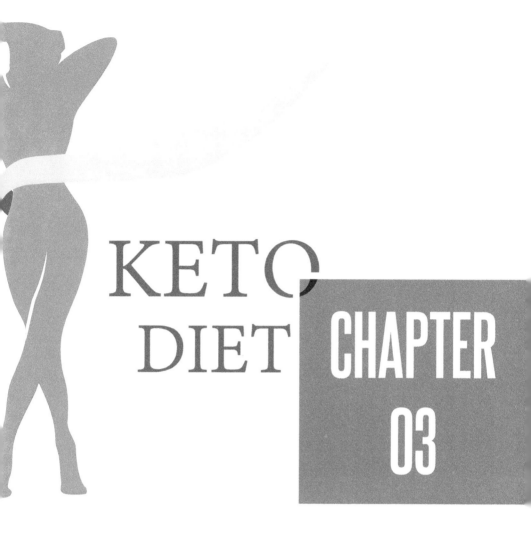

KETO DIET

CHAPTER 03

CHANGES IN YOUR BODY AFTER 50

Chapter 03-Changes in your Body After 50

For women, the biggest hormonal change that happens in menopause. Menopause is a natural part that every woman experiences as a result of their aging process.

These hormone fluctuations don't only drag unpleasant symptoms with them, but they also have a serious negative effect on other hormones as well:

INSULIN

Science has found out that decreased levels of estrogen can promote insulin resistance, and in turn, increase blood sugar. We all know that insulin is a hormone produced by the pancreas to regulate the glucose levels in our blood. When you have insulin resistance, your body is practically immune to the effects of insulin. When that happens, your cells do not open up for glucose to enter, which leaves the blood sugar endlessly traveling in the bloodstream. The pancreas then keeps producing more and more insulin to keep up with the higher glucose levels, but it is all in vain. The levels of blood sugar are elevated, and your body is resistant to insulin. This may lead to diabetes, weight gain, and many other health issues.

GHRELIN

It is known that during menopause, women experience a significant rise in the ghrelin hormone. The ghrelin hormone is also called the hunger hormone, as it stimulates the appetite and promotes the storage of body fat:

The ghrelin levels are increased. You feel hungry and trigger the reward center of the brain. Your desire for food is increased. The process of digestion speeds up and allow for calories to be absorbed much faster. The ghrelin in your gut gets released even faster.

Thanks to the rise in their ghrelin levels, women in menopause struggle with weight gain and experience an increase in abdominal fat.

These hormonal changes cause unpleasant symptoms, during, but also after the menopause transition. The decrease of estrogen may be a natural occurrence, but it puts the body through a very challenging phase of adjusting that causes mood swings, hot flashes, fatigue, insomnia, and several other fluctuations in the nervous system and brain. Some natural therapies can help women cope with these changes, but most women after 50 will tell you that maintaining weight and keeping the overall health balanced is a real struggle. The most effective way to manage the unpleasant age-related symptoms and restore the hormone balance is to rethink your diet and adopt a Ketogenic lifestyle.

Women over 50 – and those that have already been affected by menopause – besides the menopausal symptoms, in general, share three other health issues in common: low stomach acid, low thyroid function, and a sluggish gallbladder.

LOW STOMACH ACID

As we grow older, our stomach slows down the production of necessary acid, so most women that go through menopause do not have the adequate levels of acid for their stomachs to be functioning normally. This is an important issue that needs to be addressed. However, if thinking about starting a Ketogenic diet, low stomach acid should be specially regulated as it plays an essential role in the digestion of protein, as well as eliminating bad microbes.

Thankfully, regulating stomach acid isn't that tricky. Depending on the severity of your condition, you can restore your gut balance without any special supplements. Doctors say that simply squeezing lemon juice or sprinkling apple cider vinegar over your meat and veggies will help you pre-metabolize the food you consume, which will aid the process of digestion.

To boost the quality of your digestive juices, make sure to consume more fermented foods such as sauerkraut and kimchi, fermented drinks such as coconut kefir, and up the ginger intake.

Another trick that can help you improve stomach acid is to be mindful of consuming drinks during meals. Keep in mind that drinking plenty of water with meals only dilutes your digestive juices, so make sure to leave the hydration outside the meals.

Also, make sure to time your protein consumption. It is best to eat protein-rich foods at the beginning of the meal for better stomach acid support.

If your condition is more severe and these simple strategies don't do you much good, then you should probably take supplements half-way through mealtimes.

LOW THYROID FUNCTION

Thyroid dysfunctions are not a strange occurrence for women and are especially common for older women or those that have already started experiencing the menopause symptoms. Women over 50 often struggle with hypothyroidism (low function) and experience lower vitality, unstable mood, decrease in energy, and an increase in weight.

Choosing the Keto lifestyle itself should take care of the problem if your thyroid hormones are not significantly imbalanced. Burning fat for energy and depriving your body of glucose should make women more flexible metabolically and stabilizes their blood sugar, which should, in turn, support a balanced production of the thyroid hormones.

But if you are suffering from hypothyroidism, you shouldn't put all your money on this Keto benefit. If your thyroid hormones are not balanced, then you should also address this issue by making sure to consume an adequate amount of calories. If your body doesn't receive enough calories, it may go to a conservation state and experience a drop in the T3 thyroid hormone.

Those of you who are seriously struggling with hypothyroidism will benefit the most from a Ketogenic diet combined with carb cycling to increase the calorie intake.

SLUGGISH GALLBLADDER

Having a sluggish gallbladder may not seem like a particularly serious issue, but it can surely lead to many health-concerning issues. And besides, if you are willing to give the Keto diet a try, then restoring gallbladder health and bile production is a definite must. Why? Because the gallbladder is known to be the reservoir for bile, and bile being a digestive juice that helps the fat emulsion and the creation of fatty acids, you can easily connect the dots and see why it is so important when you are utilizing ketones for energy.

There are many ways in which you can improve bile production and restore your gallbladder health. Supporting the stomach acid, eating smaller meals, and staying hydrated can all do wonders for your gallbladder.

Consuming foods that are rich in chlorophyll and higher in fiber can also do the trick. Broccoli, kale sprouts, bitter herbs, and fermented foods all support gallbladder health. But perhaps the most successful natural supplement that people with sluggish gallbladder should try is MCT oil.

MCT oil is a natural product that has been refined from coconut oil. It provides a ketone source that is easy-to-digest and readily absorbed so that your liver and overall digestive tract will not have much work to do. This will relieve the stress on the gallbladder and restore its balance.

Chapter 04-Menopause

PERIMENOPAUSE

Women can start experiencing hormonal changes related to menopause, years before their menopause begins. This stage is known as perimenopause, and the average age that women enter this stage is 46, but, of course, this depends on many factors and is different for every woman.

During this stage, periods become unpredictable and less frequent, and this lasts for about 5 years. This stage lasts 6 years and ends one year after the woman's last period.

Estrogen at this stage – Dips irregularly.

MENOPAUSE

Women enter menopause when they are around 51 or 52 years old. You know you are officially in menopause if one year has passed since the last period (if some other medical condition does not cause that, that is). Although the menopause symptoms, such as night sweats and hot flashes, begin in the perimenopause stage, during actual menopause, they are at its peak in menopause stage.

Estrogen at this stage drops rapidly, causing noticeable changes such as bone loss and extreme hot flashes.

POST-MENOPAUSE

Post-menopause is the stage that occurs after menopause is considered over, which varies from woman to woman. Typically, post-menopause occurs during women's 50s. And while the menopause stage is officially finished, most of the symptoms will still be there.

Estrogen at this stage continues dropping, which causes natural changes in the body. That may cause women to continue experiencing menopause symptoms (although not so severe) such as hot flashes.

But, why does it all happen? To understand better the natural changes in your body, think of the hormones as little messengers that travel through the bloodstream and bring a dose of regulation to chemical and physical functions in our bodies. For women in their 50s, the main culprit for the change in their bodies is the ovaries.

The ovaries produce hormones that regulate the reproductive system – estrogen and progesterone. The hormones that control these two hormones are the Follicle-Stimulating Hormone (FSL) and the Luteinizing hormone (LH). At this point, we are more concerned with the FSL hormone.

The FSL hormone is the messenger that sends an order of estrogen production and contributes to the release of eggs from the ovaries. When the woman reaches a certain age and enters perimenopause, her ovaries produce a decreased amount of estrogen because the ovaries have fewer eggs than during the reproductive years. But since the FSL messenger doesn't get the memo that the release order shouldn't be sent because there aren't that many eggs, this hormone gets increased. Trying to stimulate the production of estrogen, during these years, women have a higher level of the FSH hormone in their blood.

Peri-menopausal and menopausal women often describe sudden feelings of anxiety, or of being "overwhelmed," or of feeling tearful for no reason. Others report feelings of depression, and some experience rage, again, for no obvious reason.

Estrogen is linked with the production of serotonin, one of the neurotransmitters involved in the regulation of emotions and moods.

Low serotonin is associated with low mood and confusion, high serotonin with happiness, and an increased ability to learn and carry out complex tasks. In the middle, it is calm. Very high serotonin levels result in a state similar to sedation, and very low is associated with some debilitating psychiatric conditions. Regulation of serotonin is essential for our emotional health, and most types of medication used in the treatment of depression have the effect of maintaining levels of serotonin in the blood.

Estrogen slows down the rate at which serotonin is taken out of the bloodstream and also increases the sensitivity of the brain to serotonin by increasing the number of serotonin receptors on the brain cells.

During "perimenopause," the levels of estrogen may rise sharply and then drop.

When estrogen rises, so do serotonin levels. When it crashes, serotonin levels do the same. Women are familiar with the effects of these types of changes as they are responsible for the emotional changes many of them experience just before a period, as estrogen levels drop dramatically (albeit temporarily).

So throughout the perimenopausal and menopausal stage, women may be experiencing the equivalent of random PMT.

Serotonin is not the only neurotransmitter involved in estrogen related mood swings. Estrogen also slows down the rate at which both dopamine and norepinephrine are absorbed. Low estrogen results in low levels of these neurotransmitters. Dopamine is involved in regulating mood, and our feelings of reward and pleasure. Low levels lead to depressive moods.

On the other hand, very high levels of dopamine lead to feelings of aggression, irritability, impulsivity, and, ultimately, psychosis. High levels of estrogen may keep dopamine levels too high. This explains the feelings of anger and aggression that some women experience as part of PMT - estrogen levels are at their highest just before they plummet at the end of a cycle.

Norepinephrine regulates the fight and flight response to the threat, as well as alertness and energy, and at high levels produce feelings of stress and anxiety. Break it down too fast, and we are left without energy and the capacity to respond to stressful situations. If levels build-up, we may be overcome with anxiety. Estrogen regulates the levels of norepinephrine through the same mechanism as dopamine.

As a result, during the peri-menopause, the impact of changing estrogen levels on serotonin, dopamine, and norepinephrine can result in moods that fluctuate from depression to rage.

This is, of course, the extreme. Many of us will survive with occasional feelings of anxiety or depression, and some will barely notice a difference.

What Can We Do about Mood Swings?

EXERCISE

Exercise is a great mood enhancer. Not only does it release endorphins, another group of neurotransmitters that give us a natural "high," but it also raises the levels of dopamine, norepinephrine, and serotonin. If your dipping estrogen levels are getting you down, exercise can help to redress the balance. Any form of exercise, a vigorous walk, or even climbing a flight of stairs, can help.

It may be the last thing you feel like doing when you are in a low mood, but it is the quickest way to correct your rebellious physiology. Most of us would not hesitate to take a pill, side effects, and all if it was going to make us feel better instantly. Exercise can do exactly that, and the side effects are all good.

If your mood has swung into an angry phase, the increased levels of serotonin brought about by exercise can calm you, and you can burn off the surplus energy of outrage.

Some people find it easier to take exercise in an organized form. You do not necessarily have to join a class. There are plenty of online courses, and YouTube is a great source of self-help videos. On the other hand, joining a class and getting involved may be exactly what you need - we are all different.

DIET

Eat a healthy diet. Go easy on caffeine, sugar, and alcohol, all of which may have effects both directly on mood, and indirectly on the important mood-regulating neurotransmitters.

Eating a healthy diet, low in processed foods, artificial colorings, salt, and sugar, can improve your energy levels and your general state of health, which will put you in a better state to deal with mood swings.

Diet is also important in helping to control or reduce your weight. How does this help with mood? Low self - esteem tends to creep in with menopause, as a manifestation of low mood, but also as a symptom of our concerns about aging. Staving off the middle-age spread, or shedding surplus pounds can help with this. As you lose weight, exercise, with all its mood-enhancing benefits,

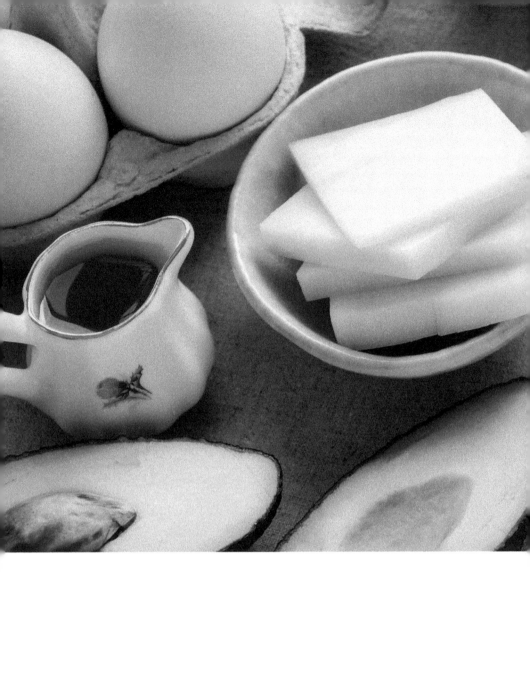

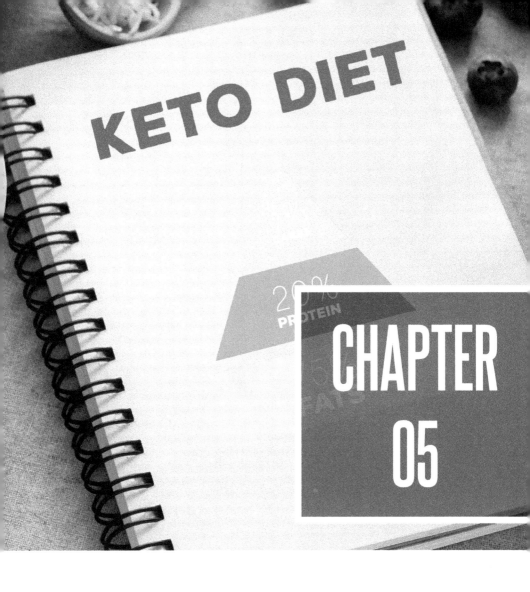

KETO DIET

BENEFITS OF KETO DIET FOR WOMEN OVER 50

Chapter 05 - Benefits of Keto Diet for Women Over 50

GGrowing older is an undeniable fact of life, but it is possible to maintain a healthy and active lifestyle long into your later years. The key to doing this is to make good choices when it comes to your health, and choosing to follow the keto diet is one of the best choices you can make. Although the keto diet is good for promoting weight loss, it has so many more benefits beyond just losing a few pounds.

One benefit of the keto diet, especially in older people, is the benefits that it offers to your brain. Following the keto diet can result in a better ability to focus and an increase in overall brain function. Your brain will normally use sugar to drive its functions, but sugar has its drawbacks and is not healthy for the rest of the body. The brain can easily adapt to using ketones for fuel and function. And since the keto diet was originally invented to help control seizures in patients with epilepsy, we know it has good effects on the brain. One important side effect of the keto diet is that it seems to reduce the risk of developing Alzheimer's disease. It is believed that Alzheimer's patients suffer from increased activity in certain parts of the brain, much like people with epilepsy do, and the low carb keto diet helps to reduce the inflammation in the cells of the brain that are responsible for these conditions. And overall cognitive function and memory are enhanced in people who consume a keto diet.

Your risk of developing some form of cardiovascular disease will be greatly reduced when you begin following the keto diet. Cardiovascular disease is any disease that strikes any part of the cardiovascular system, so this includes strokes, heart attacks, high blood pressure, high cholesterol, blood clots, plaque buildup, clogged arteries, and peripheral artery disease. Cardiovascular disease can affect your entire body in some way. Carrying excess weight will cause excess fat cells to float around in your bloodstream, and this can lead to plaque buildup. Excess weight can also cause high blood pressure and high cholesterol. Losing weight will lead to a decreased risk in developing any of the forms of cardiovascular disease, and the keto diet will help you do that by making your body use stored fat for energy, which will lead to overall weight loss.

Another benefit of the keto diet in weight loss and cardiovascular health is the fact that the keto diet depends on good fats to fuel your body. The typical diet that most people consume is overloaded with saturated fats and Trans fats. You will find these types of fats in pre-packaged snack foods, processed foods, baked goods, breaded foods, and deep-fried foods. Saturated fats and Trans fats are the fats that help to hold foods together because they become solid. Think butter;

butter is a saturated fat because it is solid. The polyunsaturated fats and monounsaturated fats of the keto diet remain in their liquid state and are much healthier for your body. You will find these good fats in olives, fatty fish, avocados, and nuts and seeds, and these are all staple foods on the keto diet. Trans fats and saturated fats are the main cause of high cholesterol and high triglycerides. Since these fats are solid, think of what they probably look like inside of your arteries.

As we age, we will fall victim to inflammation. There is good inflammation that helps your body to heal when it is injured or sick. The bad inflammation comes from a poor diet and excess weight, causing excess pressure on your muscles and joints. This is what makes your joints swell and makes getting out of bed in a difficult morning. Whenever your body feels pain, it will send signals to your brain that natural pain relief is needed, and the brain sends the inflammation to the area to help heal it. When you lose weight by using the keto diet, you will eliminate much of the inflammation that you are now feeling. And the low carb aspect of the keto diet will also help to relieve inflammation because carbs cause inflammation in your body. And when you decrease the levels of inflammation in your body, you will also help to reduce or eliminate eczema, arthritis, irritable bowel syndrome, psoriasis, and acne.

The regular consumption of excess carbs will cause the elevation of particular compounds in your body that cause gout, kidney stones, and kidney disease. These compounds are usually eliminated in the urine, but if there is more than the body can eliminate, then these compounds will build up in your body. When you first start on the keto diet, the elevated ketones will cause a similar effect, but this will level out as your body flushes toxins out of your cells. After that, the levels of these compounds in your body will dramatically decrease because they will no longer have a high consumption of carbs to fuel their growth.

A diet that is high in carbs can cause gall bladder disease, which includes gall stones and blockages. When you consume food, your liver releases cholesterol, which tells the gall bladder to release bile; so that your stomach and intestines can digest your food. If you consume too much food, your liver produces too much cholesterol, and your gall bladder produces too much bile, and the result is that it will collect, unused, inside of your gall bladder and develop gall stones. When you eat a diet that is low in carbs, you will eliminate most of the cholesterol that builds up in your body. Your body makes enough cholesterol on its own and does not require more from your diet, which it gets when you consume a diet that is high in carbs. And the high-fat consumption of the keto diet will help the gall bladder to clean itself and to keep functioning properly.

The acid levels in your stomach are increased by the consumption of processed foods, sugary foods, high carb foods, grain-based foods, and certain fruits and vegetables. This increase in stomach acid leads to acid reflux, heartburn, and eventual damage to your esophagus. Your esophagus relaxes just enough to allow food to pass down into your stomach, and the muscles of the esophagus help to begin the process of digestion as they pass the food along. The band of muscles at the bottom is supposed to tighten to prevent food from coming back up. However, after years of inflammation from high carb foods, overeating, and excess stomach acid, these muscles are weakened, and stomach acid can easily travel back up your esophagus, causing heartburn and reflux. When you consume a low carb diet, you will relieve the inflammation that occurs in the esophagus and stomach and help to ease or eliminate acid reflux and heartburn.

Probably the best good side effect of the keto diet is that it will help you to lose weight since an accumulation of excess weight is responsible for almost all of the chronic illnesses that older women suffer from. Getting rid of obesity means reducing or eliminating inflammation and metabolic syndrome, which happens when your cells stop responding to the insulin that brings food to them. Metabolic syndrome is the last stage your body experiences before the onset of Type 2 Diabetes. Following the keto diet forces, your body uses its excess fat stores for energy, and this will cause the production of insulin by your pancreas to return to normal levels. And the amounts of protein and fat you will consume on the keto diet will help you to feel fuller for longer periods so that you will not be tempted to overeat or to turn to sugary treats and processed snacks.

As women age, they may experience hair loss and brittle fingernails due to a loss of collagen and biotin. The keto diet will help with both of these issues. The increased levels of protein will provide collagen and eggs, nuts, and certain low carb veggies that will provide you with biotin.

You will eat less food on the keto diet, and that may put some people off in the beginning. It might be difficult to believe that you will be able to survive on what may seem like such a small amount of food. But the carbs you have been used to eating turn to sugar in your body, and you feel the need to eat more food to keep yourself full. The keto diet relies on the consumption of healthy fats and good proteins that will fuel your body and keep you feeling full for longer than carbs will. This will lead to a reduction in the calories that you consume, which will make you lose weight and feel better. As you lose weight and decrease the amount of inflammation in your body, you will feel better and look better. And these are how the keto diet will benefit you and improve your life.

Chapter 06 - Figure Out What to Eat

Now that we have gotten to the exciting part, it is time to learn what you can and cannot eat while following your new diet. Up until this point, you have most likely followed the food pyramid stating the importance of fruits and vegetables. While they are still going to be important for vitamins and nutrients, you are going to have to be selective. Below, you will find a complete list of foods you get to enjoy on the ketogenic diet!

KETO-FRIENDLY VEGETABLES

Vegetables can be tricky when you are first starting the ketogenic diet. Some vegetables hold more carbohydrates than others. The simple rule that you need to remember is above the ground is good; below the ground is bad — got that?

Some popular above-ground vegetables you should consider for your diet (starting from the least carbs to the most carbs) include:

- Spinach
- Lettuce

- Avocado
- Asparagus
- Olives
- Cucumber
- Tomato
- Eggplant
- Cabbage

- Zucchini
- Cauliflower
- Kale
- Green Beans
- Broccoli
- Peppers
- Brussel Sprouts

And the below-ground vegetables you should avoid include:

- Carrots
- Onion
- Parsnip
- Beetroot

- Rutabaga
- Potato
- Sweet Potato

Every food that you put on your plate is comprised of three macronutrients: fat, protein, and carbohydrates. This will be an important lesson to learn before you begin your new diet, so be sure to take your time learning how to calculate them.

The golden rule is that meat and dairy are mostly made from protein and fat. Vegetables are mostly carbohydrates. Remember that while following the ketogenic diet, less than 5% of your calories need to come from carbohydrates. This is probably one of the trickiest tasks to get down when you are first getting started; there are hidden carbs everywhere! You will be amazed at how fast 20 grams of carbs will go in a single day, much less a single meal!

When you are first getting started, you may want to dip your toes into the carb-cutting. As a rule, vegetables that have less than 5 net carbs can be eaten fairly freely. To make them a bit more ketogenic,

I suggest putting butter on your vegetables to get a source of fat into your meal.

If you still struggle at the store, figuring out which vegetables are ketogenic, look for vegetables with leaves. Vegetables that have left are typically spinach and lettuce, both that are keto-friendly. Another rule to follow is to look for green vegetables. Generally, green vegetables like green bell peppers and green cabbage are going to be lower in carbs!

KETO-FRIENDLY FRUITS

Much like with the vegetables, many berries and fruits contain hidden carbs. As a general rule, the larger the amount of fruit, the more sugar it contains; this is why fruit is seen as nature's candy! On the ketogenic diet, that is a no go. While berries are going to be okay in moderation, you should leave the other fruits out for best results.

You may be thinking to yourself; You need to eat fruits for nutrients! The truth is, you can get the same nutrients from vegetables, costing you fewer carbohydrates on the ketogenic diet. While eating some berries every once in a while won't knock you out of ketosis, it is good to see how they affect you. But, if you feel like indulging in fruit as a treat, you can try some of the following:

- Raspberries
- Cherries
- Blackberries
- Blueberries
- Strawberries
- Clementine
- Plum
- Cantaloupe
- Kiwi
- Peach

KETO-FRIENDLY MEAT

On the ketogenic diet, meat is going to become a staple for you! When you are selecting your meats, try to stick with organic, grass-fed, and unprocessed. What I do want you to keep in mind is that the ketogenic diet is not meant to be high in protein, it is meant to be high in fat. People often link the ketogenic diet to a high meat diet, and that simply is not true. As you begin your diet, there is no need to have excess amounts of meat or protein. If you do have excess protein, it is going to be converted to glucose, knocking you right out of ketosis.

There are several different proteins that you will be able to enjoy while following the ketogenic diet. When it comes to beef, you will want to try your best to stick with the fattier cuts. Some of the better cuts would include ground beef, roast, veal, and steak. If poultry is more your style, look for the darker, fattier meats. Some good options for poultry selection would be wild game, turkey, duck, quail, and good old-fashioned chicken. Other options include:

- Pork Loin
- Tenderloin
- Pork Chops
- Ham
- Bacon

On your new diet, you will also be able to enjoy several different seafood dishes! At the store, you will want to look for wild-caught sources. Some of the better options include mahi-mahi, catfish, cod, halibut, trout, sardines, salmon, tuna, and mackerel. If shellfish is more your style, you get to enjoy lobster, muscles, crab, clams, and even oysters!

Keep in mind that when selecting your meats; try to avoid the cured and processed meats. These items, such as jerky, hot dogs, salami, and pepperoni, have many artificial ingredients, additives, and unnecessary sugars that will keep you from reaching ketosis. You know the better options now, stick with them!

KETO-FRIENDLY NUTS

As you begin the ketogenic diet, there is a common misconception that you will now be able to eat as many nuts as you would like because they are high in fat. While you can enjoy a healthy serving of nuts, it is possible to go too nuts on nuts. Much like with the fruits and the vegetables, you would be surprised to learn that there are hidden carbohydrates here, too!

The lowest carb nuts you are going to find include macadamia nuts, Brazil nuts, and pecans. These are fairly low in carbohydrates and can be enjoyed freely while following the ketogenic diet. These are all great options if you are looking for a healthy, ketogenic snack or something to toss in your salad.

When you are at the shop, you will want to avoid the nuts that have been treated with glazes and sugars. All of these extra add sugar and carbohydrates, which you are going to want to avoid. The higher carb nuts include cashews, pistachios, almonds, pine, and peanuts. These nuts can be enjoyed in moderation, but it would be better to avoid.

The issue with eating nuts is that it is easy to overindulge in them. While they are technically keto-friendly, they still contain a high number of calories. With that in mind, you should only be eating when you are hungry and need energy. On the ketogenic diet, you will want to avoid snacking between meals. You don't need the nuts, but they taste good! If you want to lose weight, put the nuts down, and stick to a healthier snack instead.

KETO-FRIENDLY SNACKS

On the topic of snacks, let's take a look at keto-friendly ones to have instead of a handful of nuts! Before we begin, keep in mind that if you are looking to lose weight, you will want to avoid snacking when possible. In the beginning, it may be tougher, but as you adapt to the keto diet, your meals should keep your hunger at bay for much longer.

If you are looking for something small to take the edge off your hunger pangs, look for easy whole foods, some of these basics would include eggs, cheese, cold cuts, avocados, and even olives. As long as you have these basics in your fridge, it should stop you from reaching for the high-carb foods.

If you are looking for a snack with more of a crunch, vegetable sticks are always a great option! There are plenty of dipping sauces to add fat to your meal, as well. On top of that, pork rinds are a delicious, zero-carb treat. Beef jerky is also a good option, as long as you are aware of how many carbohydrates are in a commercial package.

With the good options in mind, it's always good to take a look at the bad. When you are snacking, avoid the high-carb fruits, the coffee with creamer, and the sugar-juices. Before you started the ketogenic diet, these were probably the easy option. You'll also want to avoid the obvious candy, chips, and donuts. Just remember when you are selecting your foods, ask if it is fueling you or not.

Keto-Friendly Oils, Sauces, and Fats

On the ketogenic diet, the key to getting enough fat into your diet is going to depend on the sauces and oils you use with your cooking. When you put enough fat into your meals, this is what is going to keep you satisfied after every meal. The secret here is to be careful with the labels. You may be surprised to learn that some of your favorite condiments may have hidden sugars (looking at you, ketchup.)

While you are going to have to be a bit more careful about your condiments, you can never go wrong with butter! Up until this point, you have probably been encouraged to consume a low-fat diet. Now, I want you to embrace the fat! You can put butter in absolutely anything! Put butter on your vegetables, stick it in your coffee, and get creative!

Oils, on the other hand, can be a bit more complicated. You see, natural oils such as fish oil, sesame oil, almond oil, ghee, pure olive oil, and even peanut oil can be used on absolutely anything. What you want to avoid are the oils that have been created in the past sixty years or so. The oils you'll want to avoid include soy oil, corn oil, sunflower oil, and any vegetable oil. Unfortunately, these oils have been highly processed and may hinder your process.

Stick with these for your diet instead:

- Butter
- Vinaigrette
- Coconut Oil
- Mayo
- Ranch Dip
- Mustard
- Guacamole
- Heavy Cream
- Thousand Island Dressing
- Salsa
- Blue Cheese Dressing
- Ranch Dip
- Pesto

When it comes to dairy, high fat is going to be your best option. Cheese and butter are great options but keep the yogurts in moderation. When it comes to milk, you will want to avoid that as there is extra sugar in milk. If you enjoy heavy cream, this can be excellent for your cooking but should be used sparingly in your coffee.

Keto-Friendly Beverages

Remember that staying hydrated, especially when you are first starting your new diet, is going to be vital! Your safest bet is to always stick with water. Whether you like your water sparkling or flat, this is always going to be a zero-carb option. If you are struggling with a headache or the keto fly, remember that you can always throw a dash of salt in there.

Chapter 07 - Get your Body into Ketosis and Become Fat Adapted

Keto-adaptation is the process in which your metabolism shifts from depending on glucose to relying mainly on fats as a source of energy. As oxidation of fats increases, your body also begins to produce ketone bodies to serve as an alternative source of fuel. Fat oxidation involves the breakdown of fats into free fatty acids. These free fatty acids are then broken down further in the liver to form ketone bodies.

The free fatty acids can be used as an energy source by almost every tissue in the body except the nervous system and brain. This is why they have to be broken down further to form ketones. The nervous system and brain need ketones to work efficiently in the absence of glucose.

This whole process of transitioning from glucose to fats and ketones does not happen overnight. Your metabolism needs some time to adjust to the new diet and energy source. You may begin to see some changes in your body within a couple of days of following the Ketogenic diet, but the adaptation process itself takes weeks.

During keto-adaptation, you will experience a delay between when you first reduce your carbohydrate consumption and having an efficient fat-burning metabolism. During this period, you will feel sick (also known as keto-flu), slow and fatigued.

- Keto-flu tends to mimic the symptoms of regular flu

It is important to keep your carb intake low during keto-adaptation; otherwise, your body will not adapt as it should. Most people either give up or cheat by eating more carbs, but this will interfere with ketosis, and you will simply be prolonging the process.

There are steps you can take to minimize those initial negative effects of keto-adaptation. For now, let's look at why keto-adaptation is important and how carbohydrates interfere with the process.

THE SELF-PERPETUATING CYCLE

One of the first things you must realize is that the more carbs you consume, the more dependent you become on glucose as a source of energy. The problem with glucose is that it is utilized so fast by the body that it leaves you hungry again within a short time. As you eat more carbs to replenish your stocks, you delay your body's ability to adapt to fat-burning. But where and how does this cycle start?

Your body can store only a very small amount of glucose, and this is done in the form of glycogen. There are two types of glycogen in the body: muscle glycogen and liver glycogen. Your liver can only store about 100 grams of glycogen while your muscles can store about 400 grams. However, the use of muscle glycogen is restricted only to the muscle that stores glycogen. For example, the glycogen in your bicep muscle can only be used by the tissues in your bicep. In other words, muscle glycogen cannot re-enter the bloodstream and travel somewhere else.

This means that liver glycogen is the only source that the body can use to stabilize your blood sugar and provide fuel for your brain. Remember that you only have 100 grams to work with, and this is a very small amount that cannot get you through the day. If your body has not yet adapted to making use of ketones for energy, you must find a way to replenish your liver glycogen. Otherwise, you will feel mentally and physically fatigued.

Estimated Energy Stores in Humans

There are two ways to get more glucose into the bloodstream. Option 1 is to eat some carbs, continue being dependent on glucose, and prevent your body from utilizing alternative sources of fuel. If you do this, you will find it very difficult to adapt to ketosis, and the negative side effects of the initial stages will be prolonged.

Option 2 is to allow your body to manufacture glucose from protein in a process known as gluconeogenesis. This process is why it is not necessary to eat carbohydrates to get glucose. The body can make its glucose in small amounts from protein, much the same way that Vitamin D is manufactured naturally by exposure to sunlight.

In other words, when you feel tired and hungry, you don't need to grab a carbohydrate meal. A lot of fats, moderate protein, and very little carbs are enough to help you make it through the day. Even after your liver glycogen runs out, there's no need to worry because your body will resort to gluconeogenesis and then ketosis to provide fuel for your needs.

One of the things you will notice during keto-adaptation is that you won't feel like eating or snacking as often as you did before. You will be able to skip meals and not feel as hungry. A Ketogenic diet can help you naturally balance your blood sugar without becoming a slave to carbohydrates.

PHASES OF KETO-ADAPTATION

Keto-adaptation generally occurs in three stages:

1.   INITIAL PHASE

During this first phase of keto-adaptation, your body will still be dependent on liver glycogen. The initial phase is very tough for most people because, to break the self-perpetuating cycle, you must stop eating carbohydrates. During this first phase, your liver glycogen stores will be dwindling, metabolism of fat will still be sub-optimal, and ketone production will be insignificant. It is safe to say that you will experience a lot of fatigue and brain fog during the first three days to two weeks.

Then there is the water loss. One aspect of the storage of glycogen is that it requires much water. Research shows that every gram of glycogen in the body requires about 3 or 4 grams of water to be stored with it. This means that as glycogen stores are depleted, you may end up losing a maximum of 2 kilograms of water! On top of that, high insulin levels usually cause water retention in the body.

Since a low-carb diet reduces insulin levels around the body, excess water can then be excreted. Therefore, you will experience drastic weight loss within the first few weeks of the Ketogenic diet.

Initially, the weight loss will primarily be excess water

However, there is one critical thing to note here. Even though you will lose water-weight during the initial phase, this will gradually decrease, and you will soon begin to lose actual fat as keto-adaptation progresses.

2. ADJUSTMENT PHASE

In this second phase, your glycogen stores will have been depleted, and your body will now start making ketone bodies. Some of these ketones will be released through the urine and can be measured easily using the method described. This will enable you to confirm that you have achieved the right level of carbohydrate restriction. This phase usually takes between six and eight weeks.

During this phase, ketones are freely available as an energy source, but the levels are not yet stable enough. At this point, something quite interesting happens in the brain and muscles in regards to ketone use. When the levels of ketone bodies are still low, the muscles utilize them directly as a source of fuel, but as the levels increase, the muscles suddenly utilize them less and instead switch to fat as a fuel source. The brain, on the other hand, utilizes ketones according to their proportion in the bloodstream. When ketone levels are low, the brain only uses a small amount that allows it to function, but when ketone levels rise above a specific threshold, supply to the brain rapidly increases.

Now that there is enough supply of energy, the brain can be fully dependent on ketones, since there is no risk of running out of fuel. Your brain doesn't need you to eat frequently to work optimally, while your muscles now depend on fat to supply energy. This aspect of keto-adaptation is the one that athletes find quite valuable.

3. MAINTENANCE PHASE

In this phase, your body has adapted to ketosis. The maintenance phase simply involves making the Ketogenic diet a lifestyle, and this may take up to a year or two of consistently keeping your carbs low. The aim here is to make it a habit and continue reaping the benefits for a long time to come.

MAKING KETO-ADAPTATION EASIER

It is clear to see that the initial phase of keto-adaptation can be very difficult to handle for two specific reasons. The first reason is that there is very little glucose left and not enough ketone and fat metabolism to provide energy. Therefore, the best way to cope is to consume a large amount of fat. Even though your ultimate goal is to utilize body fat for energy, you must still get much fat from your diet, especially during the initial phase.

The fat will provide your body with essential nutrients and fatty acids which are needed for producing energy. You should know by now that there is nothing to fear by eating a lot of dietary fats, so long as they're the right kind of fats.

- Start by gradually increasing your intake of healthy fats

The second reason is that your body is losing a lot of water, sodium, and potassium at a very fast rate. This is responsible for fatigue, headaches, and weakness. Make sure that you consume enough sodium every day. Take about five grams or two teaspoons of table salt daily to avert these symptoms.

- Table salt will help avert fatigue and headaches during keto-adaptation

You will need to get enough potassium and magnesium to prevent loss of lean muscle, cramps, dizziness, and fatigue. Meat is a good source of these minerals, but make sure that you preserve the water if you boil your meat. Potassium and magnesium tend to dissolve when meat is boiled, so use the water to make some broth.

- Beef broth is a great source of mineral salts

You can also take mineral supplements to help prevent any acute effects. It is also very important that you don't forget to drink a lot of water.

- Potassium and magnesium supplements will help you adapt better to ketosis

You should also ensure that you consume very little carbohydrates. If you start experimenting with your carb tolerance level at this stage, you will fail to adapt to ketosis. Make sure that you know just how much carbs your food contains. Choose a very low carb intake level (about 20 grams per day) and commit to it for as long as possible until your body starts to produce ketones. Once you know how much to eat, stick to it if you want to achieve total keto-adaptation.

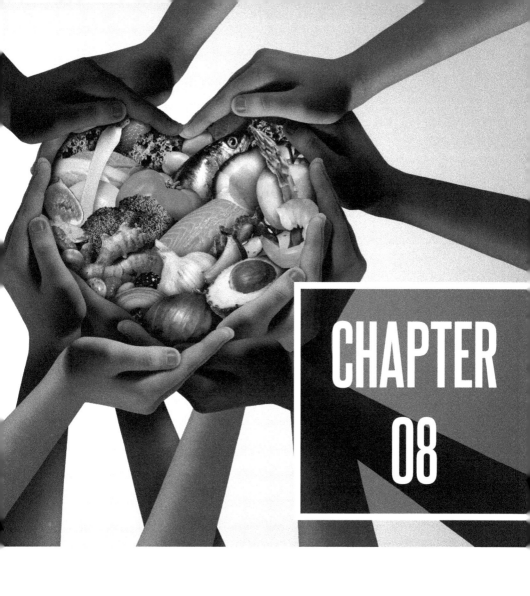

CHAPTER 08

HOW TO HAVE MORE ENERGY ?

Chapter 08 - How to Have More Energy?

If feeling worn out seems to be a regular pattern in your life nowadays, this is yet another reason why trying the Keto diet can benefit you. Everyone deals with their stressors and tasks throughout the day, but the way that the body handles all of this can differ greatly. Your food is your fuel, so it makes sense that what you put into your body is super important for making it through each day. Most of us tend to feel completely drained by the end of a long day, but this doesn't have to be your standard way of feeling. When you put the right fuel into your body, it will create more energy than you've ever had before.

Keto can provide you with energy that lasts, not fleeting bursts. When you only receive energy in bursts, from coffee or sugar, for example, this creates the eventual feeling of a crash. This happens because the energy is only meant to be temporary and while it can get you through a moment, it isn't going to carry you throughout your whole day. The energy that Keto can give you is the more permanent energy. It is the kind of energy that builds up gradually, preventing you from ever feeling like you are going to crash.

In the Standard American Diet (SAD), carbs are overconsumed. In general, American's eat too many simple carbs and unhealthy fats. Most of the time, the carb takes the center of the plate, with a side of protein, and little, if any, healthy fats. Additionally, we are junk food junkies - we eat too many processed foods that are often high in carbs and sugars, eat sugared "health" foods, like sugary/syrupy yogurt, and eat out at restaurants that dish out huge servings, loaded with terrible fats, a ton of carbohydrates. Because of this high intake of the wrong kind of carbs, these starches will be converted into glucose or sugar molecules.

Based on your knowledge of how the body works while it is not on a Keto diet, you can gather that your body is simply going to absorb the glucose and then use that for energy. This is where the fleeting energy problem becomes very real. In order to complete this process, your body needs insulin. As your glucose levels rise, so will your insulin. Even when your body has had enough, it continues to store the extra energy (glucose) for later. The insulin will also send your body signals to your liver that the glucose stores are now full. Assuming that your body is not insulin sensitive or insulin resistant, everything should go well.

As you age, though, your body can change in a way that will make it less able to handle its insulin levels properly. When your body realizes that it needs to catch up, it will demand itself to work even harder. Sometimes, it just isn't possible for it to do so. This is when you will find that many problems arise. You might find that you have unnecessary glucose in your bloodstream. If your body isn't burning it, then it simply collects until it gets the message to do something with it. During these periods, you will likely have your biggest surges of energy. However, these are the kind that can make you very tired after only a few hours later. These spurts of energy are ultimately not useful in the long run.

It is when your body's energy levels experience these drops that you begin feeling sluggish and start to crave more sugar and carbs. Since that is what you originally gave your body for this energy that you are receiving, it is naturally going to crave more of it. If you aren't careful, this can lead to unhealthy snacking and eating habits. You might find that you are craving quick snacks to get your fix and this usually means that you are going to reach for processed or artificial foods. You do not need to have insulin resistance to experience this. It is just the way that you are training your body by the diet that you are deciding to eat.

If you feel that you can identify with these energy highs and lows, you are not alone. So many people feel this way all the time, but they do not know how to tailor their diet to truly change the pattern. For most, adjusting the carbs that are consumed is not enough. This is when you will begin to feel hungry and cranky. Eating fewer carbs without replacing them is simply telling your body that you are giving it less fuel. This will begin an internal resistance that will likely leave you feeling frustrated. At the end of the day, you will probably still want to reach for those junk food favorites.

Keto is a way for you to ensure that you are properly replacing your carbs. When you follow a Keto diet based on the given percentages, you should be getting everything that you need to keep your energy levels steady. There should be no highs and lows, only medians that you will be able to reach. By receiving energy in this way, your body isn't going to think that this is the only energy it will receive for the day. Therefore, it will not go into a state of overworking, followed by a big crash. Keto is all about balance and that is the one thing to keep in mind when you are seeking more energy.

Those who make the switch have expressed their concerns, much like concerns that you probably have. A lot of people worry that Keto just won't be enough to sustain them. They anticipate a lot of snacking and binge eating to correct this, but then they are pleasantly surprised when they realize that there is far less snacking needed throughout the day. When you can let go of the stigmas that surround the diet, you will find that your body will go through a natural process of adjustment. When you are changing anything, you need to make sure that you commit to the change.

The Keto diet does drain all of your energy stores, but it replaces them with healthy fats. A lot of people assume that Keto is bad for you because it is like you are starving yourself, but that is not how it works. You are simply changing the way that your body operates and how it utilizes this energy. Your body isn't going to be angry with you for this switch like you might expect it to be. While it is an adjustment, your body is going to quickly realize that it can tap into the extra energy stores for more fuel whenever it needs to. It will learn what to do with these healthy fats that you are providing and how to make them last for long periods.

You will be able to say goodbye to your afternoon slumps and instead feel that you have enough energy to power through any day. There is also less of a chance that you will feel grumpy or "hangry" in-between meals. Typically, when you are between meals, your body is waiting for you to give it more energy. Since your body stores this energy when you are on a Keto diet, there are reserves for it to dip into, which truly allow you to experience your day without feeling like you are being distracted by hunger or cravings. Know that your transition into the Keto diet is going to vary. Depending on how carb-heavy your current diet is, it might take your body some time to retrain itself. For most people, it happens fairly quickly, though. You might have to deal with a few days of an unsettled stomach before you truly begin to experience the benefits of Keto, but it should not be enough to deter you.

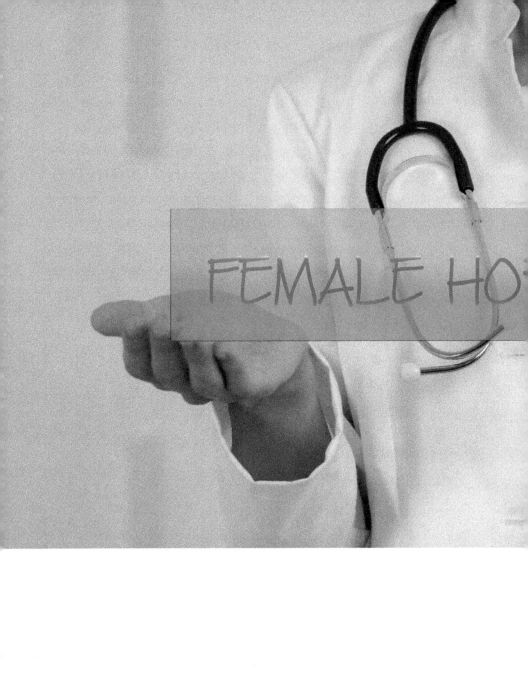

CHAPTER 09

HORMONE BALANCE

Chapter 09 - Hormone Balance

With a more thorough understanding of how the ketogenic diet can help balance your hormones, it is time to learn how! By embracing the ketogenic life and applying these lessons to your everyday life, you will enjoy this diet in no time. Remember that while it will take some extra effort at first, it will be thoroughly worth it. The first thing you will want to do is focus on your diet! One of the most beneficial steps you can take is starting eating foods rich in probiotics. By doing this, you will keep your gut bacteria in check. Also, plan to eat more protein for about three days before your period, to help keep your hormones in check.

Another way you can help your hormone balance is to eat foods rich in calcium. Foods such as almonds, salmon, celery, sesame, and poppy can help with symptoms that are associated with mood swings. If you ever have questions, you can always test your hormone levels to make sure they are in check. The ones you will want to pay special attention to include cortisol, progesterone, estrogen, and SBHG. While this isn't diet-related, managing your stress levels is a vital part of balancing your hormones. Remember that stress had a major effect on your hormones, so you need to address the issue at hand. To help combat stress, remember to move your body, sleep well, and spend time with your loved ones.

Finally, you will want to test your pH levels. As we age, maintaining the alkalinity within your diet will be key. Alkalinity has a direct effect on your vitamin absorption, lowers inflammation, improved bone density, and helps you maintain a healthy weight. Luckily on the ketogenic diet, you will balance this in your diet.

ALKALINE KETOGENIC DIET

You are already well aware of what the ketogenic diet is, but what is an alkaline diet? We base this dieting around eating acidic foods that alter your pH balance. As you eat, your metabolism breaks down the food into metabolic waste through chemical reactions. The metabolic waste is acidic (pH under 7.0), neutral (pH of 7.0), or is alkaline (pH over 7.0). According to the alkaline diet, the pH of your metabolic waste influences your body's acidity. When your body is too acidic, this leads to health issues such as heart disease, cancer, diabetes, hypertension, and osteoporosis. To improve the acidity of your body, create an alkaline state in your body through diet.

When you create an alkaline environment in your body through the ketogenic diet, you will experience incredible benefits such as lowering inflammation within the body, balancing your hormones, and slow down the aging process. An alkaline diet can also help support your overall health by reducing the symptoms often in association with infertility, menopause, and PMS.

Your body is naturally alkaline. Depending on what you eat can heighten or lower your pH balance. Much like with testing ketones, you can test your pH balance through a urine testing kit. In an ideal world, you want to strive for a pH between 7.0 and 7.5. The question is, how?

The answer you are looking for is the ketogenic diet. When you combine an alkaline diet with a low-carb diet, you are lowering the number of toxic substances you are sticking in your body and providing it with more nutrients through your new diet.

To further your process, fasting is another way to keep yourself healthy and allows your body the time to take a break from the function of digesting. By doing this, your body has time to repair other parts of you and can send its energy toward helping the cells rather than digesting your dinner!

With all of this in mind, note that the ketogenic diet, while beneficial, may not completely solve your issues. Other problems can cause hormonal issues such as hypo/hyperthyroidism, over-training, stress, not eating enough, and other pre-existing hormonal balances. If you continue to struggle with your hormones, get checked out by a professional. As earlier said, there are benefits to the ketogenic diet, but it will not cure you by magic. With that being said, if it doesn't help your hormone balance, which does not mean that you will not experience others, enjoys your new diet; stick with it!

Ketosis is the ultimate goal of the ketogenic diet. It's defined as a metabolic state of greater ketone production and enhanced fat burning. But it also comes with a plethora of health benefits. For women; however, Ketosis apparently triggers a range of unpleasant side effects.

A properly executed ketogenic diet can help to restore the balance to out-of-whack female sex hormones. In my practice, I've also seen it mitigates weight gain, hot flashes, near-zero energy, low sex drive, bone loss, mood swings, and other troublesome symptoms associated with perimenopause, menopause, PMS, and post-menopause. Women who are going through major homone changes or dealing with symptoms related to homone flunctuation. I employ ketogenic nutrition to help them fix their hormones and keep them feeling healthy; especially, as they get older. Here's how and why the ketogenic diet can come to your rescue:

1. It focuses on fat for better hormone support.

Fat is your best friend on a ketogenic diet. On a true keto diet, roughly 75 percent of your calories should come from healthy fat sources; such as, avocados, nuts and seeds, coconut oil, butter, olives and olive oil, and other high-fat foods. These "good" fats support hormone production and maintain hormone balance because they are the building blocks for estrogen, progesterone, and testosterone. For too long, we've been told to be wary of fat, and thus we slashed fat in favor of carbs. This was a mistake, and personally; I believe that, this low-fat movement contributed to the hormonal challenges that many women face today.

2. It boosts insulin sensitivity by reducing carb intake.

A keto diet restricts carbohydrates from 20 to 50 grams a day. This helps balance insulin levels. Insulin is a master hormone that controls blood sugar, and when it's too high and out of balance, your sex hormone levels can drop.

Luckily, following a ketogenic diet makes your body more "insulin sensitive." This means insulin is well-regulated, in balance, and used properly by your cells. When you're insulin sensitive, all sorts of metabolic miracles happen. You stay slim and get fit more easily; you lower your risk of cardiovascular disease, Alzheimer's disease, and dementia; you tend not to have hot flashes or night sweats; and you rebuild your bone health so that you're less at risk for frailty and osteoporosis. Cravings become a distant memory, and you feel and look healthy and energized.

3. It eases premenstrual syndrome (PMS) by detoxing the body.

PMS produces a lot of really uncomfortable symptoms, including cramps, cravings, moodiness, irritability, depression, acne, and fatigue. The underlying cause is often estrogen dominance, or having too much estrogen and not enough progesterone. One of the causes of estrogen dominance is a diet comprised of too much sugar and refined carbohydrates — a problem easily eliminated by going on a ketogenic diet.

Another cause of estrogen dominance is exposure to estrogens in the environment. These are toxic forms of estrogen that not only worsen PMS symptoms, but they are through; to increase the risk of breast cancer, endometriosis, infertility, and autoimmune diseases. In my version of a keto diet, you're encouraged to eat foods that detoxify these nasty estrogens like veggies such as broccoli, cauliflower, Brussels sprouts, cabbage, and greens and delicious herbs and spices like oregano, thyme, rosemary, sage, and turmeric.

4. It boosts reproductive health by combating PCOS.

One of the main causes of infertility in women is polycystic ovary syndrome, or PCOS. This condition develops from poorly balanced sex hormones, and more than half of the women diagnosed with PCOS are obese or overweight, have poor blood sugar regulation, and have insulin resistance. There's no cure for PCOS, but because insulin problems are associated with PCOS, a ketogenic diet is a viable solution. Duke University researchers found that women with PCOS who followed a keto diet were able to balance their levels of insulin and testosterone and experience improvements in weight, infertility, and menstruation among other factors. Two women in the study got pregnant despite infertility problems, and everyone lost weight.

5. It zaps stress to protect the adrenals.

In response to life's many stressors, the adrenal glands release the hormone cortisol to galvanize energy so we can react quickly to whatever challenge we're facing. If our stress goes unresolved, the adrenals keep pumping out cortisol, resulting in too much cortisol floating around. The ongoing secretion of high amounts of cortisol robs your body of progesterone, estrogen, and testosterone, and if this keeps happening, you're more likely to experience imbalanced sex hormones, high blood sugar, loss of muscle, low sex drive, and burnout.

To combat this, enjoy all those low-carbohydrate vegetables you typically eat on a ketogenic diet (plenty of green leafy vegetables, parsley, kale, beet greens, broccoli, cauliflower, and so forth). They may help normalize cortisol, support your adrenal glands, and improve your natural progesterone levels.

The keto diet isn't for everyone, but for a lot of women in my practice it's been a game-changer for hormonal imbalance and hormone-related symptoms. If you're suffering or just not feeling your best, the keto diet is definitely worth a try!

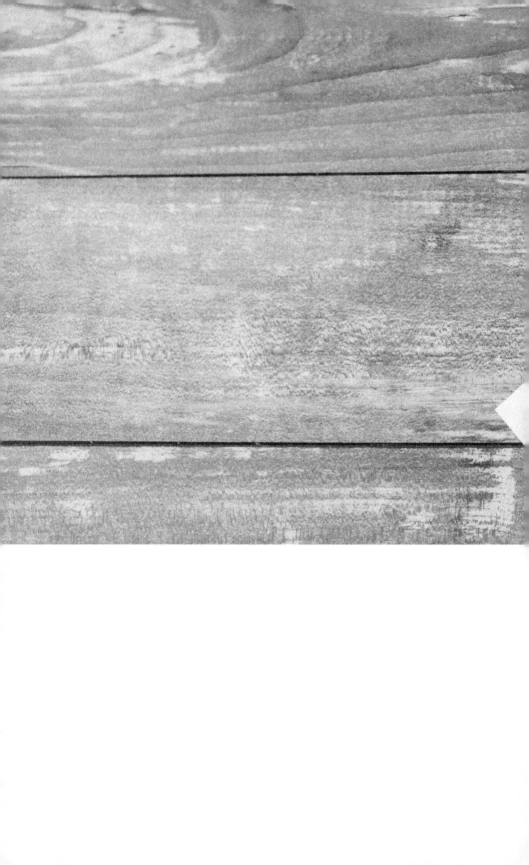

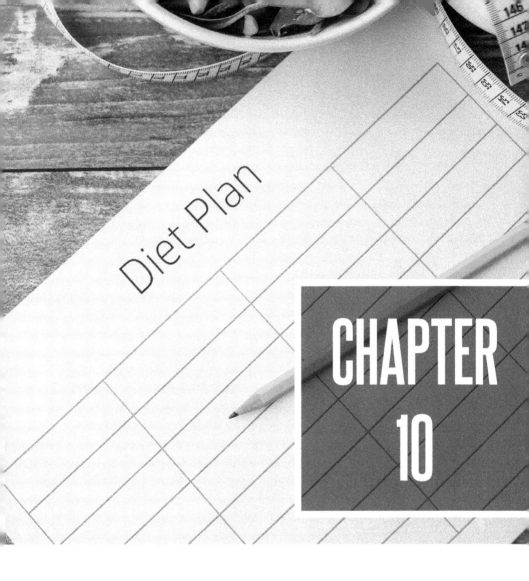

KETO DIET NUTRITION.
30 DAY MEAL PLAN

Chapter 10 - Keto Diet Nutrition. 30 Day Meal Plan

This contains a 30-day meal plan for Keto Diet to help you eat the right amount of food and keep track of daily intake. Also, to avoid the food, you should not eat in Keto diet. The meal plan will help you save a lot of time since your meal is already planned and avoids wasting food. Furthermore, the meal plan saves you a lot of money and refrain you from eating outside. The meal plan provides you a nutritionally well-balanced meal throughout the week. Meal from breakfast, lunch, dinner, and snack is provided for your convenience.

Day	Breakfast	Lunch	Dinner	Snack
1	Bacon Cheeseburger Waffles	Green Beans Salad	Korma Curry	Keto Cheesecakes
2	Keto Breakfast Cheesecake	Apple Salad	Zucchini Bars	Keto Brownies
3	Egg-Crust Pizza	Asian Salad	Mushroom Soup	Raspberry and Coconut
4	Breakfast Roll-Ups	Octopus Salad	Stuffed Portobello Mushrooms	Chocolate Pudding Delight
5	Basic Opie Rolls	Shrimp Salad	Lettuce Salad	Peanut Butter Fudge
6	Almond Coconut Egg Wraps	Lamb Salad	Onion Soup	Cinnamon Streusel Egg Loaf

7	Bacon & Avocado Omelet	Coconut Soup	Asparagus Salad	Snickerdoodle Muffins
8	Bacon & Cheese Frittata	Broccoli Soup	Beef with Cabbage Noodles	Yogurt and Strawberry Bowl
9	Bacon & Egg Breakfast Muffins	Simple Tomato Soup	Roast Beef and Mozzarella Plate	Sweet Cinnamon Muffin
10	Bacon Hash	Green Soup	Beef and Broccoli	Nutty Muffins
11	Bagels With Cheese	Sausage and Peppers Soup	Garlic Herb Beef Roast	Pumpkin and Cream Cheese Cup
12	Baked Apples	Avocado Soup	Sprouts Stir-fry with Kale, Broccoli, and Beef	Berries in Yogurt Cream
13	Baked Eggs In The Avocado	Avocado and Bacon Soup	Beef and Vegetable Skillet	Pumpkin Pie Mug Cake

14	Banana Pancakes	Roasted Bell Peppers Soup	Beef, Pepper and Green Beans Stir-fry	Chocolate and Strawberry Crepe
15	Breakfast Skillet	Spicy Bacon Soup	Cheesy Meatloaf	Blackberry and Coconut Flour Cupcake
16	Brunch BLT Wrap	Taco Stuffed Avocados	Roast Beef and Vegetable Plate	Keto Cheesecakes
17	Korma Curry	Buffalo Shrimp Lettuce Wraps	Breakfast Roll-Ups	Keto Brownies
18	Zucchini Bars	Keto Bacon Sushi	Basic Opie Rolls	Raspberry and Coconut
19	Mushroom Soup	Keto Burger Fat Bombs	Almond Coconut Egg Wraps	Chocolate Pudding Delight
20	Stuffed Portobello Mushrooms	Caprese Zoodles	Bacon & Avocado Omelet	Peanut Butter Fudge

21	Lettuce Salad	Zucchini Sushi	Bacon & Cheese Frittata	Cinnamon Streusel Egg Loaf
22	Onion Soup	Asian Chicken Lettuce Wraps	Bacon & Egg Breakfast Muffins	Snickerdoodle Muffins
23	Asparagus Salad	Prosciutto and Mozzarella Bomb	Bacon Hash	Yogurt and Strawberry Bowl
24	Beef with Cabbage Noodles	Ketofied Chick-Fil-A-style Chicken	Bagels With Cheese	Sweet Cinnamon Muffin
25	Roast Beef and Mozzarella Plate	Cheeseburger Tomatoes	Baked Apples	Nutty Muffins
26	Beef and Broccoli	Green Beans Salad	Baked Eggs In The Avocado	Pumpkin and Cream Cheese Cup
27	Garlic Herb Beef Roast	Apple Salad	Banana Pancakes	Berries in Yogurt Cream

28	Sprouts Stir-fry with Kale, Broccoli, and Beef	Asian Salad	Breakfast Skillet	Pumpkin Pie Mug Cake
29	Beef and Vegetable Skillet	Octopus Salad	Breakfast Roll-Ups	Chocolate and Strawberry Crepe
30	Beef, Pepper and Green Beans Stir-fry	Shrimp Salad	Basic Opie Rolls	Blackberry and Coconut Flour Cupcake

Capter 11 - How to Follow the Diet at Home and Away from Home

Everyone on the keto diet knows that the most available foods are not keto-friendly. There are so many foods out there that are rich in carbs but contain lots of preservatives, processed sugar, and other things that harm our body. This is one of the reasons why it's so easy to get fat. A Keto diet for the road might seem impossible, but it can be done. To help you, here are some tips you can stick to when on a keto diet, even on the road.

EAT WELL BEFORE DEPARTING

Before going out, make sure you take enough of your favorite low-carb food. Don't get all too excited or in a hurry to get started on traveling. Just make sure you get enough of your fill before setting on the journey.

KEEP SNACKS HANDY

This is an important aspect of the keto diet, you should know. Even though the keto diet keeps you energized all day and keeps you from being hungry for several hours, it is essential to keep a keto-friendly snack around when going on a journey. Nuts, hard-boiled eggs, and beef jerky are some examples of snacks you can keep around for the journey. It is generally important to have a starch of keto-friendly snacks at home, at work, or in your car because you never know when you might need them.

Some of my favorites include:

• Mixed nuts

• Hard-boiled eggs (you can get this from grocery or convenience stores).

• You can also get bags of turkey/Salmon jerky/beef/chicken. However, check the sugar before buying it

• You can get sting cheese, cheese pack, or sliced cheese

• Avocados — you can make a snack of your own by sprinkling salt on it for a satisfying and delicious snack

• Canned sardine can also make a delicious keto-friendly snack

• Any type of pre-cooked meat – This takes some time of planning. Rather than grilling up some burgers for your dinner, try grilling some and then wrap them in a foil to take with you

• Boxed salad and dressing – This is a quick way to get some greens. You can add it with your grilled meat for a perfect lunch

• Peanut or almond butter and cut celery

All you have to do is just to come up with ideas for different foods and snacks that are keto-friendly. All that is important is to have something to eat on the go without any fuss. This can be essentially important when everyone eats something on the journey and you don't want to feel left out.

PRE-MADE LUNCHES

The importance of pre-made lunches cannot be overemphasized. You can make it super-fancy or just simple. One of the keys to successful dieting is pre-made lunches. As with the above where you get to grill some meats, you could do the same, and buy a box of salad and dressing. You can eat them for the entire week. You can just add avocado, cucumber, hard-boiled eggs, mushrooms, or salted asparagus, and any seasonal vegetables. You can add something to make it feel like a gourmet, such as beef jerky. Make sure to check that your salad dressing does not contain lots of carbs or sugar (ranch, oil vinegar, blue cheese can also work).

Other nice options are:

- Celery and bun-less cheeseburgers and dressing

- Grilled Portobello mushrooms and chicken thighs

- Tuna salad lettuce cups

- Keto-friendly sandwiches — meat, bacon, cheese, avocado, and mustard between red lettuce or romaine

Fast food options and Eating out

Many people often complain that their keto diet makes it difficult to eat out, but this is not so true. You can eat out by simply cutting out the carbs. For instance, ordering a burger or sandwich which comes with chips or French fries. You can substitute lettuce for buns or rather, you can ask for it to be served on a bed of greens. You can also request salad instead of taters. Although some restaurants might sell the salad to you, it's just a little price to pay to stick to your diet.

For breakfast, you can do the same. You can substitute salad for toast in addition to your omelet. Instead of hash browns, you can request sautéed or grilled vegetables. And for dinner, you can replace bread with lettuce and substitute all the starch with vegetables.

When traveling and you make the stop to get some food in a restaurant, you probably know already that many places are better at serving burgers on top of lettuce or with lettuce buns. If the restaurant doesn't take the buns out of the sandwich, you can simply take it off yourself. Make sure you avoid chicken nuggets because they certainly contain carbs and are not keto-friendly.

Cheat days

It is not advisable to cheat on your diet more than once in a week, but at least you are allowed to cheat sometimes on a trip. This is one of the best parts of the keto diet; it lets you cheat now and then as far as you get back to it as quickly as possible. So in times of a night out with some friends for some pizza and beer, you can go ahead. In the morning, be prepared to get back on your diet. As far as you do it, your body will be back in ketosis soon enough.

LEARN TO FAST

Fasting is one of the most difficult parts of the keto diet, but it remains a very effective aspect. If you are just getting started on a keto diet, fasting is not yet suitable for you. In the beginning, you just have to pay attention to getting enough to eat so you won't be super hungry.

As you stick to the diet, with time, you will notice you are not as hungry as you used to be. At this point, you can start fasting. An easy way to fast is to make use of the time you are sleeping as a starting point. When morning comes, get a coffee and in the middle of the day, you can treat yourself to a little snack like some nuts and hard-boiled eggs. You can fast with your snacks the next day. After that, you can wait until lunch before having a whole meal. With this, you have fasted for 42 hours, which is not bad.

Several pieces of research showed many benefits of intermittent fasting. Even if all you can do is fast for just 15 to 20 hours, it's still enough. The best time length for fasting for health purposes is three days. It is believed that fasting for this duration several times in a year helps to prevent cancer.

The best thing about the fast is that you don't have to treat it as a serious fast more than once a month, especially a moment you get into the rotation of 15 to 20 hours fast now and then. If you are used to eating three to four times per day, you will have a lot of work on your hands. However, if you can learn to fast, then it will be a powerful tool that can help you achieve your goal.

Chapter 12 - How to Keep Track of your Keto Diet

Keeping track of your Keto diet is something that is important and will go a long way towards your success. The first thing that you have probably noticed is that the eBook has already talked a little about tracking what you are doing with measuring your ketones. This is something that is important, but there is so much more to the diet than just eliminating carbs and increasing your protein and high-fat content. This is, unfortunately, an oversimplification of the diet, but that's the bad news, the good news is when you keep track of the diet you will be able to discern the relationships between the different types of food that you are consuming and how it affects not just how you get into the state of ketosis but how you feel when you eat these foods. The goal of the diet is for you to lose weight and feel great, so if you are losing weight but you are not feeling great, then something is wrong, and it needs to be fixed so that it why tracking what you are doing is so very important. Make sure that you are detailed in your tracking of what you do so that you can be sure that you are getting the most out of your Keto Diet. Focusing on things like the percentages along with the foods you ate and what times is a great place to start.

Naturally, there are questions about how to track your progress, but the good news is the techniques that are out there for tracking your progress come down to repetition and being detailed. The more you can add, the better you will do. Now, before we get into a longer discussion about the things to track and how to track them, what you need to know is that there are a ton of apps out there that will help you keep track of your progress on the Keto Diet and help you make sure that you are not straying outside the lines with how you are working your specific ration. The good news is that these apps can go on your smartphone, and you can carry them around with you to have you in a better position for making sure that you are sticking with your diet. There are a few things that are important to track, though, and they are signposts for how well you are doing on the Keto Diet.

WEIGHT LOSS

The most important thing that you can track with the Keto Diet is your weight loss. This is the critical component of the diet and the ultimate end goal. There are several ways that you can track your weight loss, but the first thing you need to do is get a scale. The good news is you do not need a scale that does all sorts of things like measure body fat and whatnot; instead, you can get a scale that will simply display your weight. These scales are relatively cheap and are at every single major store.

Once you have your scale, the next thing to do is weigh yourself. The key to weighing yourself is to do so every single day at the same time and under the same circumstances. The best way to track your weight is to weigh yourself in the morning when you wake up, but after you have gone to the bathroom. This is when you are at your most accurate weight because your body has gotten rid of most of its excess weight. Check your weight. There are several things to do here. You could record your weight on the app that you chose to track your progress on the Keto Diet, or you could keep a chart. One really helpful thing is the social promotion aspect of how you are losing weight. Posting your weight every day on social media will get people that are in your life to rally around you and provide encouragement. It also helps you stay on top of your game. The last thing that you want is to be in a position where you want to get out of the diet. So keeping track of your weight is especially important because it ensures that you are sticking with the diet and making sure the diet is doing exactly what you need it to do – keeping you healthy and losing weight.

As you use the programs to track your weight, track other changes as well. Take your measurements. What is your waist size and your chest size? This is where bad fat gets stored, so if you know what your size is. You do your measurements every couple weeks, and this is another way to give yourself the positive reinforcement you need to make sure that you are doing what needs to be done to lose the weight and keep it off when getting on the Keto Diet.

Tracking your Food

This is something else that is important – you have to keep track of what you eat with the Keto Diet. This matters because as you eat the food, you are also going to be testing your levels of ketones in your body. When you do a food diary, this is a great way to make sure that you are doing the right levels of calories along with the different grams of food that you need to eat. There are so many different things to do with a food diary, but when you keep a food diary, what ends up happening is that you can correlate how you are feeling and your levels of ketones with what you are eating. This, in turn, makes your time on the Keto Diet that much more productive – you can lose weight with greater efficiency, and in turn that make it so that you can easily keep yourself faithful to the diet. Having a food journal is easy to do, and it is found on many of the Keto Diet apps.

Tracking your Ketones

The other thing that people on the Keto Diet need to do is stay abreast of where their numbers are. Now when it comes to testing yourself, doing stuff like taking a blood test is something that you should not do every day because you will not see much variance. However, if you want to make sure that each day you are doing a little bit better, it is very easy to use the tools such as the breath analyzer and the urine strips. These tools make it so easy to check your levels of ketones, see if you are in ketosis, and at the end of the day, make sure that you are doing what is necessary to keep yourself in this state in conjunction with the food that you are eating and the substances you are drinking.

That being said, the initial foray into ketosis is not the easiest thing, so that requires a lot of patience. With all of the different Keto Diet apps that are out there, you can be sure to input the readings, and some of the different devices are even able to integrate with the apps, which makes them that much more formidable when it comes to keeping track of all the different things that you are doing. The bottom line is that as long as you are getting the numbers that you need to see and that they are heading in the right direction, you can rest assured that it will be quite simple to get to the point where your body is burning your fat cells instead of looking for the different glycogen stores – because those glycogen stores are not there.

When it comes to tracking what you do, it is always better to be disciplined and vigilant with your tracking. This is the simplest way to make sure that what you are doing is producing results. The worst thing would be if you are trying to keep track of stuff, but at the same time, you are not able to correlate the data with the outcomes. The Keto Diet does require a massive amount of cohesion with all of the different elements, and that is why this is not the easiest of diets, but when you are keeping track of everything that you are doing, what ends up happening is that the diet becomes a rewarding endeavor and the signposts that you get from the tracking are things that keep you engaged with the diet and pushing yourself to greater heights for weighing that you can lose along with being that much more healthy. So, find a Keto Diet app that you like and get started right away with tracking all the different parts of the diet.

Chapter 13 - Tips on Losing Weight on Keto After 50

EXERCISE

In the fitness world, it is already established that 80% of your weight loss success comes from the diet. So just by following the keto diet alone, you are already making great progress. However, if you want that extra edge in your weight loss, consider doing exercises.

You have plenty of options here. You can do cardio exercises such as jogging, running, or cycling every morning for 30 minutes, but strength training works just as well for older adults. You should do both if you can.

Cardio exercises can get the heart pumping and get the body moving more freely, but note that your muscle mass starts to decline after 50. So work on your muscles as well.

How much exercise should you do? It depends on how much you can handle. No point in pushing beyond the limit and regret it later, right?

TEAM UP

A group activity is always more entertaining. So if you can find like-minded individuals who are also into keto diets, consider doing it together with them. It makes things much easier. This tip also applies to some other tips that I will show you, such as the exercise that I just covered.

MOVE MORE

Moving more here does not mean more cardio exercises. You cannot expect to get any more effective weight loss if you exercise for 30mns a day and then sit on the couch for the rest of the day. The idea is to burn more calories than you can take in, so it pays to be a little extra active throughout the day.

If you have a desk job, consider getting up at least once an hour and take a short break by walking in the lobby for at least 5 minutes. It doesn't seem much, but it helps in the long run.

MORE PROTEIN

Protein is very important for both weight loss and youth, including the protection against muscle degradation and other aging ailments.

Couple a high protein intake with strength exercise, and you can be sure that you would be building muscles faster than they can degrade. You won't look like Arnold when he was a bodybuilder, but you might even look fitter than the guy in his 20s at your workplace.

Talk to a Dietitian

The first thing you should do before getting into any diet is to consult your dietitian. While the keto diet works for many people, you never really know if it will work for you. Therefore, it is wise to ask your dietitian first before you jump in, rather than suffer some adverse effects because your body is not compatible with this diet.

Cook at Home More

Or eat out less frequently. There are two reasons why you should do that. For one, there are only a few places, if at all, that serve keto-based foods, let alone those that follow your diet plan. You need to prepare your food if you want to do a keto diet. Another benefit is economics. You will buy most of your ingredients and prepare your meals ahead of time. This means you will only spend your money on the ingredients you know you will need.

Eat More Produce

While we are on the subject of eating, consider incorporating more produces in your diet, some of which I have covered already. Vegetables and fruits are full of nutrients that your body needs to remain healthy, so it should be included in your diet.

HIRE A PERSONAL TRAINER

While we are still discussing exercising, consider getting yourself a personal trainer. That way, you can get the most out of your exercises, and your trainer also doubles as an exercise partner as well because they hold you accountable for your commitments. Your trainer is very helpful when you do strength training because they can teach you how to perform the exercise with the correct form and to prevent you from injuring yourself.

RELY LESS ON CONVENIENCE FOODS

Convenient foods are convenient but not healthy. Not by a long shot. They are rich in calories and often do not pack essential nutrients such as protein, fiber, vitamins, etc. If you can, ditch inconvenient foods altogether.

FIND AN ACTIVITY YOU ENJOY

When you have done enough exercise, you will know what activities you like. One way to encourage yourself to exercise more regularly is by making it entertaining than a chore. If possible, stick to your favorite activities, and you can get the most out of your exercises. Keep in mind that the activities you enjoy may not be effective or needed, so you need to find other exercises to compensate, which you may not enjoy so much. For instance, if you like jogging, then you can work your leg muscles, but your arms are not involved. So you need to do pushups or other strength training exercises.

Here, your trainer can help you decide and create a workout routine that you can stick with as well.

CHECK WITH A HEALTHCARE PROVIDER

As mentioned earlier, the keto diet works for many people, but it isn't for everyone. Your dietitian can tell you whether the keto diet would work. However, it helps to check in with your healthcare provider to ensure that you do not have any medical condition that prevents you from losing weight, such as hypothyroidism and polycystic ovarian syndrome. It helps to know well in advance whether your body is even capable of losing fat in the first place before you commit and see no result, right?

EAT LESS AT NIGHT

While the science still argues about it to this day, it seems more logical that breakfast is the most important meal of the day considering that you would not have eaten for the past 8 hours whereas the interval between breakfast and lunch, and lunch and dinner is 5 or 6 hours at best. Dinner should be small because your body does not need to expend that much energy when you are sleeping anyway. So the excess energy becomes fat.

So keep dinner light. For one, it helps you lose weight. Another reason is if you have a heavy dinner, your body will strain itself trying to digest everything. That means your body would remain active until all the food is digested, meaning that you will not get restful sleep if you can sleep at all.

Bottom line: Eat light and eat dinner at least 4 hours before bedtime. Any sooner and you will have a hard time sleeping.

BODY COMPOSITION

Your body isn't just "weight" alone. Your body is composed of fat, muscles, fluid, bones, etc. What you want to lose is fat weight, not muscle weight or fluid weight. You want as little fat mass in your body as possible while still maintaining a healthy level of non-fat mass in your body. There are many ways you can measure your body fat, but the simplest method is to measure your calves, thighs, waist, chest, and biceps.

HYDRATE PROPERLY

That means drinking enough water or herbal tea and ditch sweetened beverages or other drinks that contain sugar altogether. Making the transition will be difficult for the first few weeks, but your body will be thanking you for it. There is nothing healthier than good old plain water, and the recommended amount is 2 gallons a day. However, because you are on a keto diet, your body needs to use up more water, so consider 2 gallons to the absolute minimum amount of water you need to drinks. I recommend you drink between 3 or even 4 gallons a day when you are on a keto diet. If you get thirsty, then it is a sign of dehydration, so drink some water. Drinking plenty of water also leads to additional calories burned. You can shave off a few more calories by drinking cold water because your body will spend more energy trying to regulate your body temperature.

SUPPLEMENTS

When you get older, your body starts to lose its ability to absorb certain nutrients, which leads to deficits. For example, vitamin B12 and folate are some of the most common nutrients that people over 50 lack. They have an impact on your mood, energy level, and weight loss rate.

Therefore, if you feel tired when you are on your keto diet, perhaps you do not get enough nutrients that your body needs. That does not mean you should eat more, no. You just need to take the right supplements.

GET ENOUGH SLEEP

When you are over 50, your body starts to fail you. You no longer have the ability to party past midnight without feeling horrible for the rest of the month. If there is the most crucial time to get 8 hours of sleep a day, then it is right now.

Getting enough sleep helps your body regulate the hormones in your body, so try to aim for 7 to 9 hours of sleep a day. You can get more restful sleep by creating a nighttime routine that involves not looking at a computer, phone, or TV screen for at least 1 hour before bed. You can drink warm milk or water to help your body relax or even do 10 to 20 minutes of stretching so you can get a restful sleep.

While we are on the subject of sleeping, try to maintain a consistent sleeping schedule. I understand that you want to sleep and wake up 1 to 4 hours later than usual during the weekend. But you want to go to bed and wake up at the same time, your mood and energy level will be higher. An added benefit is that your body will learn to wake up on its own even without the alarm.

MINDFUL EATING

Mindfulness isn't restricted to meditation alone. Again, we will not go over meditation in this guidebook because it is another topic altogether. But what you can do here is learn to love and appreciate your food. It sounds obnoxious, but it helps your mood and promotes weight loss.

Simply put, you just have to put away your phone and take away any other sources of distractions and focus solely on your food, how it tastes, etc. That means eating slowly. You will learn to appreciate how tasty your food is because you focus on eating.

How does this translate to weight loss? You see, there is a system in your body that determines how full you are. The issue here is that this system is not instantaneous. It takes some time to measure how full your stomach is before sending the signal to your brain. So when you eat too quickly, by the time you feel full, you would have already overshot by a country mile. If you eat slowly, your body has enough time to register your fullness bite by bite. So when you feel full, you have not overeaten.

KETOGENIC
DIET

 5% 20% 75%
PROTEIN

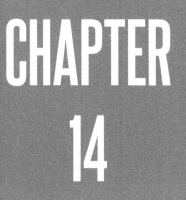

CHAPTER
14

CONCLUSION

Chapter 14 - Conclusion

Now that you are familiar with the Keto diet on many levels, you should feel confident in your ability to start your own Keto journey. This diet plan isn't going to hinder you or limit you, so do your best to keep this in mind as you begin changing your lifestyle and adjusting your eating habits. Packed with good fats and plenty of protein, your body is going to go through a transformation as it works to see these things as energy. Before you know it, your body will have an automatically accessible reserve that you can utilize at any time. Whether you need a boost of energy first thing in the morning or a second wind to keep you going throughout the day, this will already be inside of you.

As you take care of yourself through the next few years, you can feel great knowing that the Keto diet aligns with the anti-aging lifestyle that you seek. Not only does it keep you looking great and feeling younger, but it also acts as a preventative barrier from various ailments and conditions. The body tends to weaken as you age, but Keto helps to keep a shield up in front of it by giving you plenty of opportunities to burn energy and create muscle mass. Instead of taking the things that you need to feel great, Keto only takes what you have in abundance. This is how you will always end up feeling your best each day.

Arguably one of the best diets around, Keto keeps you feeling so great because you have many meal options! There is no shortage of delicious and filling meals that you can eat while you are on any of the Keto diet plans. You can even take this diet with you as you eat out at restaurants and friends' houses. As long as you can remember the simple guidelines, you should have no problems staying on track with Keto. Cravings become almost non-existent as your body works to change the way it digests. Instead of relying on glucose in your bloodstream, your body switches focus. It begins using fat as soon as you reach the state of ketosis that you are aiming for. The best part is, you do not have to do anything other than eating within your fat/protein/carb percentages. Your body will do the rest on its own.

Because this is a way that your body can properly function for long periods, Keto is proven to be more than a simple fad diet. Originating with a medical background for helping epilepsy patients, the Keto diet has been tried and tested for decades. Many successful studies align with the knowledge that Keto works. Whether you are trying to be on a diet for a month or a year, both are just as healthy for you. Keto is an adjustment, but it is one that will continue benefiting you for as long as you can keep it up. Good luck on your journey ahead!

ALICE HARWING

KETO DIET
AFTER 50

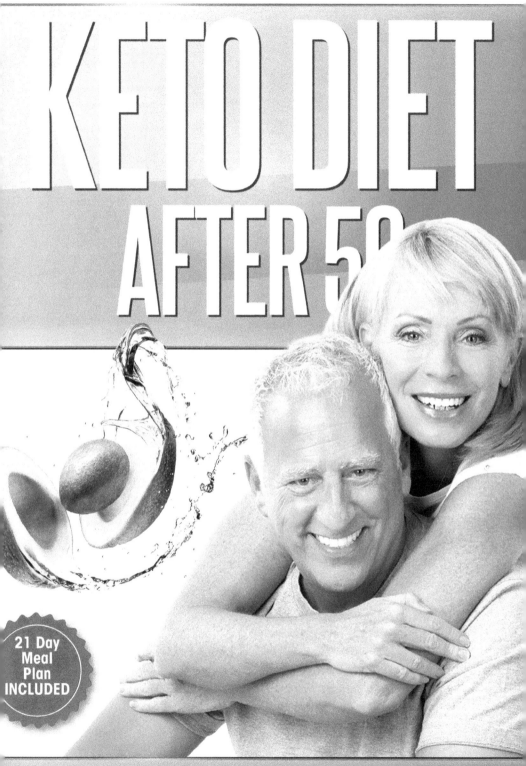

21 Day Meal Plan INCLUDED

A Feasible Approach To Have A Better Metabolism, Burn Fat,
Lose Weight, Prevent Diabetes, Get Body Confidence, Boost Your
Energy And Learn A Tasty Meal Plan

KETO DIET AFTER 50

A feasible approach to have a better metabolism, burn fat, lose weight, prevent diabetes, get body confidence, boost your energy and learn a tasty meal plan

ALICE HARWING

v

Introduction

The **Keto Diet is an** eating plan that recommends a reduction of carbohydrates in favor of higher fat intake. The Keto Diet aims to replace sugars with fats as a source of energy in the body.

The health benefits of the Keto Diet are vast. Some benefits include:

• Improved cardiovascular function

• Reduced risk of various diseases like heart disease

• Enhanced cognitive function

• Weight loss

• Decreased inflammation and oxidative stress

• Stabilized and healthier blood sugar and blood lipid balance

Well, the Keto Diet is very clear that one should eat as few carbs as possible. The best answer to this question is that the viable limits for carbs should be between 30 to 100 grams per day. Eating more than 100 grams per day will affect Ketosis.

If you are sure that what you are eating is keto-friendly, there is no need to track your macros. In short, you should not concern yourself with tracking macros if you are eating all foods listed as keto foods. However, you are supposed to track macros if you want to stray from keto foods for a snack or one meal.

Even as the Keto diet may be self-sufficient in providing the body with the required nutrients, supplements can be taken to boost certain deficiencies. However, supplements should be taken with prior consultation and approval of a dietician. Note that an abnormal intake of some supplements can cause enormous effects on the body.

Scientifically, your body can survive without consuming any dietary carbohydrates. Therefore, it is not unhealthy to forgo carbs and instead eat more fat with some protein. These two macros can healthily substitute for carbs. Remember that the main use of carbs in the body is energy production, which can be replaced by Ketosis (use of fats for energy production).

You must have heard that Ketosis is dangerous, especially to keto beginners. Well, it is not dangerous! One may just develop minor systems caused by the keto flu as the body becomes adapted to the Keto Diet. For some people, the flu is usually gone by the end of the first week. However, if the flu prolongs, it cannot go for more than three weeks.

Some people experience short-lived irritability, frequent urination, dehydration, and keto flu. After a short period, the body gets used to a low-carb and high-fat intake.

It is because your body's metabolism is experiencing dietary changes. Nothing serious, though! You just have to be patient for some time (not more than two weeks). Additionally, you can take some energy supplements such as MCT oils and exogenous ketones.

The only thing you should do is reduce your alcohol intake and know the type of alcohol to consume. Do not forget that most alcoholic drinks are very rich in carbs and unfriendly to the Keto Diet. The best option for you is pure spirits in moderate quantities. In addition, do not mix spirits with soda or fruit juices because the net effect will be adding to your carb intake.

The Keto Diet is not for everyone. It is generally better for people who want to lose weight, improve cognitive function, reduce risks of certain diseases, and enhance endurance, among other personal goals.

Chapter 01 - The Main Features of Ketogenic Diet

Losing weight: for most people, this is the foremost benefit of switching to keto! Their previous diet method may have stalled for them or they were noticing weight creeping back on. With keto, studies have shown that people have been able to follow this diet and relay fewer hunger pangs and suppressed appetite while losing weight at the same time! You are minimizing your carbohydrate intake, which means fewer blood sugar spikes. Often, those fluctuations in blood sugar levels make you feel more hungry and prone to snacking in between meals. Instead, by guiding the body towards ketosis, you are eating a more fulfilling diet of fat and protein and harnessing energy from ketone molecules instead of glucose. Studies show that low-carb diets are very effective in reducing visceral fat (the fat you commonly see around the abdomen that increases as you become obese). This reduces your risk of obesity and improves your health in the long run.

Reduce the Risk of Type 2 Diabetes: The problem with carbohydrates is how unstable they make blood sugar levels. This can be very dangerous for people who have diabetes or are pre-diabetic because of unstable blood sugar levels or family history. Keto is a great option because of the minimal intake of carbohydrates it requires. Instead, you are harnessing most of your calories from fat or protein, which will not cause blood sugar spikes and ultimately less pressured the pancreas to secrete insulin. Many studies have found that diabetes patients who followed the keto diet lost more weight and ultimately reduced their fasting glucose levels. This is monumental news for patients who have unstable blood sugar levels or are hoping to avoid or reduce their diabetes medication intake.

Improve cardiovascular risk symptoms to overall lower your chances of having heart disease: Most people assume that following keto that is so high in fat content has to increase your risk of coronary heart disease or heart attack. But the research proves otherwise! Research shows that switching to keto can lower your blood pressure, increase your HDL good cholesterol, and reduce your triglyceride fatty acid levels. That's because the fats you are consuming on keto are healthy and high-quality fats, so they reverse many unhealthy symptoms of heart disease. They boost your "good" HDL cholesterol numbers and decrease your "bad" LDL cholesterol numbers. It also decreases the level of triglyceride fatty acids in the bloodstream. A top-level of these can lead to stroke, heart attack, or premature death. And what are the top levels of fatty acids linked to?

High Consumption of Carbohydrates: With the keto diet, you are drastically cutting your intake of carbohydrates to improve fatty acid levels and improve other risk factors. A 2018 study on the keto diet found that it can improve 22 out of 26 risk factors for cardiovascular heart disease! These factors can be very important to some people, especially those who have a history of heart disease in their family.

Increases the Body's Energy Levels: Let's briefly compare the difference between the glucose molecules synthesized from a high carbohydrate intake versus ketones produced on the keto diet. The liver makes ketones and use fat molecules you already stored. This makes them much more energy-rich and a lasting source of fuel compared to glucose, a simple sugar molecule. These ketones can give you a burst of energy physically and mentally, allowing you to have greater focus, clarity, and attention to detail.

Decreases inflammation in the body: Inflammation on its own is a natural response by the body's immune system, but when it becomes uncontrollable, it can lead to an array of health problems, some severe, and some minor. The health concerns include acne, autoimmune conditions, arthritis, psoriasis, irritable bowel syndrome, and even acne and eczema. Often, removing sugars and carbohydrates from your diet can help patients of these diseases avoid flare-ups - and the delightful news is keto does just that! A 2008 research study found that keto decreased a blood marker linked to high inflammation in the body by nearly 40%. This is glorious news for people who may suffer from inflammatory disease and want to change their diet to see improvement.

Increases Your Mental Functioning Level: As we elaborated earlier, the energy-rich ketones can boost the body's physical and mental levels of alertness. Research has shown that keto is a much better energy source for the brain than simple sugar glucose molecules are. With nearly 75% of your diet coming from healthy fats, the brain's neural cells and mitochondria have a better source of energy to function at the highest level. Some studies have tested patients on the keto diet and found they had higher cognitive functioning, better memory recall, and were less susceptible to memory loss. The keto diet can even decrease the occurrence of migraines, which can be very detrimental to patients.

The Calorie and Nutrient Balance: Do you know why else the Ketogenic Diet is good for you, specifically, as someone who just hit 50 years of age? What you should keep in mind is that as a person advances in age, their calorie needs decrease. For example, instead of 2,000 calories per day – you'll need only 1,800 calories per day. Why is that? Well, when we start to age –our physical activity significantly decreases. Hence, we don't need as much energy in our system. However, that doesn't mean our nutrient needs also go down. We still need the same amount of vitamins and minerals.

The Ketogenic Diet manages to hit a balance between these two needs. You get high nutrition for every calorie you get – which means that you'll maintain a decent amount of weight without really feeling less energetic for day to day activities.

Heart Diseases: Keto diets help women over 50 to shed those extra pounds. Reducing any amount of weight greatly reduces the chances of a heart attack or any other heart complications. Through the carefully selected diet routine, not only are you losing weight and enjoying scrumptious meals, but you are significantly boosting your heart's health and reviving yourself from the otherwise dull state that you may have been in before.

Diabetes Control: Needless to say, the careful selection of ingredients, when cooked together, provide rich nutrients, free from any processed or harmful contents such as sugar. Add to that the fact that keto automatically controls your insulin levels. The result is a glucose level that is always under control, and continued control would lead to a day where you will say goodbye to the medications you might be taking for diabetes.

Chapter 02 - Benefits of the Keto Diet for People Over 50

Everyone gradually gets older. It is an undeniable fact of life. But even though we are aging all the time, we do not need to be old, not yet anyway. It is possible to be an active, vibrant woman at fifty and beyond if you make some smart choices and take care of yourself. And deciding to follow the keto way of life is the smartest choice you could have made. The keto diet isn't just good for weight loss, although that is probably its most important and noticeable feature. The keto diet gives so much more to your body while it is helping you to lose and then maintain your weight.

The keto diet will result in increased brain function and the ability to focus. The brain normally uses sugar to fuel its processes, but the consumption of sugar has its problems. The brain can easily switch to using ketones for fuel and energy. Remember that ketones are the by-product of Ketosis that makes you burn fat. And the keto diet was used by doctors to control seizures in patients long before medications were invented. The exact way this works is still not completely understood.

However, researchers believe it has something to do with the neurons stabilizing as excess sugar is removed from the diet, and hormones are better regulated. Patients with Alzheimer's disease have been seen to have increased cognitive function and enhanced memory when they consume a keto diet. And these same changes in the chemical makeup of the brain can lead to fewer migraines overall and less severe migraines.

When the keto diet helps you to lose weight, it also helps you to reduce your risk of cardiovascular disease. These diseases include anything that pertains to the cardiovascular system, which means heart attacks, strokes, plaque formations, peripheral artery disease, blood clots, and high blood pressure. Plaque buildups, which are caused by excess weight and cholesterol, lead to a condition known as atherosclerosis. The plaque will gather in the arteries and form clogs that narrow the artery and restrict the flow of blood. The plaque is formed from fat cells, waste products, and calcium deposits that are found floating in the blood. When you lose weight and decrease the amount of fat and cholesterol in the body, there will be less to accumulate in the arteries, and the blood will naturally flow better with less restriction.

Being overweight can cause high blood pressure. When the doctor measures the force of your blood pressure as it moves through your arteries, he measures your blood pressure. If you are overweight, your heart will need to push the blood harder to get it through the increased lengths of arteries, it had to create to feed your cells. And if there is a buildup of plaque in the arteries, then the heart will need to push the blood harder to get it past the blockage. This, in turn, creates thin spots in the arteries, which is a good place for plaque to build up. Since this condition comes on gradually over the course of years as you slowly gain weight, it gives off no immediate symptoms, and that is why it is often referred to as the silent killer. Strokes and heart attacks are caused by unchecked high blood pressure.

The single most important way to control high blood pressure is to control your weight. You can't change the family history, but you can control your weight and your lifestyle. Since high blood pressure is caused by the heart needing to work harder than the act reducing the strain on the heart will cause it to work less strenuously in bad ways. Losing weight and maintaining a healthy weight will ease the strain on your heart. If the blood pressure is not pumping too high, then it will not cause weak spots in your arteries. If there are no weak spots, then there is no place for plaque to collect. And if there is no excess fat or cholesterol in the blood, there will be no plaque formations to collect in the blood.

A diet that is high in saturated fats is a risk factor for heart disease. While keto is a high-fat diet, it is high in monounsaturated fats. Polyunsaturated and monounsaturated fats are good for you, while trans fats and saturated fats are not. Mono – and polyunsaturated fats are the good fats that are found in fatty fish like salmon and in certain plants like avocados, olives, and certain seeds and nuts that are all staples of the keto diet. Saturated fats and trans fats are found in breaded deep-fried foods, baked goods, processed foods, and pre-packaged snack foods like popcorn. When your doctor measures your LDL and HDL, he also measures your level of triglycerides, which is a type of fat that is found floating in the bloodstream, and that is responsible for elevating the risk of heart attacks, especially in women over fifty. Reducing the number of saturated fats and trans fats that you consume will automatically reduce the amounts of triglycerides floating in your blood.

Inflammation is a part of life, especially for women over the age of fifty. There are good kinds of inflammation, such as when white blood cells rush to a particular body area to kill an infection. But mostly older women are plagued by the bad forms of inflammation, which make your joints swell and cause early morning stiffness. Carrying too much weight on your body will cause inflammation and pain in the joints, especially in the lower part of the body where the weight-bearing joints like the knees and the hips are located. When a joint feels pain, it sends a signal to the brain that there is a pain, and the body sends cells to combat that pain. The helper cells don't know there isn't anything wrong, but they come prepared to fight, and this causes inflammation around the joint. One extra pound of excess weight will put four pounds of pressure on the knee joints. Losing weight will help to eliminate inflammation in the body. And cutting down on the intake of carbs will help to lessen the amount of inflammation in the body because carbs can cause this effect. Decreasing the inflammation in your body will also help to eliminate acne, eczema, arthritis, psoriasis, and irritable bowel syndrome.

Adopting the keto way of life will also help to eliminate problems with the kidneys and improve their function. Kidney stones and gout are caused mainly by the elevation of certain chemicals in the urine that helps to create uric acid, which is what we eliminate in the bathroom. The excess consumption of carbohydrates and sugar will lead to a buildup of calcium and phosphorus in your urine. This buildup of excess chemicals can cause kidney stones and gout. When your ketones begin to raise, the acid in your urine will briefly increase as your body begins to eliminate all of the waste products from the fats that are being metabolized. However, after that, the level will decrease and will remain lower than before as long as you are on the keto diet.

Eating a diet that is high carb can eventually cause problems with your gallbladder, including gallstones. These stones are little deposits of hardened fluid that get trapped in your gallbladder and cause great pain. The gallbladder is built to release bile into the small intestine to help digest the food that you eat. When the liver produces more cholesterol than your gallbladder can produce bile to digest, the excess cholesterol forms stones in the gallbladder. Eating a low carb diet will eliminate much of the excess cholesterol that your liver produces, and the high fat of the keto diet will help the gallbladder to cleanse itself.

Vegetables that grow in the ground, grain-based foods, processed foods, and sugary foods all contribute to heartburn and acid reflux by raising the level of acid in the stomach. There is a band of muscles that is wound tightly around the bottom of your esophagus, the muscular tube that takes food from your mouth to your stomach. This band of muscles is called the esophageal sphincter. It will relax just enough to let food pass into the stomach when it is healthy. But a constant diet of the wrong kinds of foods will increase the stomach acid, which in turn washes over this sphincter and eventually weakens it, which allows stomach acid to flow backward and up into the esophagus. Eating the low carb keto diet will improve the acid reflux symptoms and will help to relieve the inflammation of the esophagus and the stomach.

The best overall benefit of the keto lifestyle is the fact that it will lower your overall weight, which will have a positive effect on your entire body. Lower weight will mean freedom from the effects of obesity, which can help to get rid of metabolic syndrome and Type

2 Diabetes. The condition known as metabolic syndrome happens when the body becomes resistant to insulin, and the insulin your body produces is no recognized by the cells in your body. This is what causes the body to store your excess blood sugar as fat in your body, especially around the area of the stomach. When you begin the keto diet and enter Ketosis, the body will be forced to use these fat stores for energy, and the body's production of insulin will be returned to normal. The amount of protein in the diet will help your muscles keep their strength and tone and not begin to wither as so often happens in older women.

Following the keto diet will mean that you will eat less food, but it will be more filling and more nutritious. When you eat fats and proteins instead of carbs, you will feel fuller much longer with less food. Lowering your caloric intake will help you lose weight, and less weight will make you healthier. It will also slash your risk of developing certain diseases and will minimize the effects of others. These are the life improvements that the keto lifestyle has to offer you.

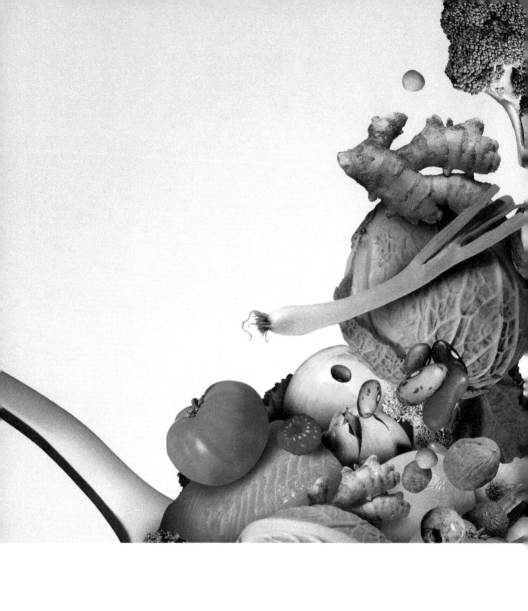

CHAPTER 03

KNOW WHAT FOODS YOU'LLL EAT AND AVOID ON THE KETOGENIC DIET

Chapter 03 - Know What Foods You'll Eat and Avoid On the Ketogenic Diet

I've had people complain about the difficulty of switching their grocery list to one that's Ketogenic-friendly. The fact is that food is expensive – and most of the food you have in your fridge is probably packed full of carbohydrates. This is why if you're committing to a Ketogenic Diet, you need to do a clean sweep. That's right – everything that's packed with carbohydrates should be identified and set aside to make sure you're not eating more than you should. You can donate them to a charity before going out and buying your new Keto-friendly shopping list.

Seafood

Seafood means fish like sardines, mackerel, and wild salmon. It's also a good idea to add some shrimp, tuna, mussels, and crab into your diet. This is going to be a tad expensive, but worth it in the long run. What's the common denominator in all these food items? The secret is omega-3 fatty acids, which are credited for lots of health benefits. You want to add food rich in omega-3 fatty acids in your diet.

LOW-CARB VEGETABLES

Not all vegetables are good for you when it comes to the Ketogenic Diet. The vegetable choices should be limited to those with low carbohydrate counts. Pack up your cart with items like spinach, eggplant, arugula, broccoli, and cauliflower. You can also put in bell peppers, cabbage, celery, kale, Brussels sprouts, mushrooms, zucchini, and fennel.

So what's in them? Well, aside from the fact that they're low-carb, these vegetables also contain loads of fiber, which makes digestion easier. Of course, there's also the presence of vitamins, minerals, antioxidants, and various other nutrients that you need for day to day life. Which ones should you avoid? Steer clear of the starch-packed vegetables like carrots, turnips, and beets. As a rule, you go for the vegetables that are green and leafy.

FRUITS LOW IN SUGAR

During an episode of sugar-craving, it's usually a good idea to pick low-sugar fruit items. Believe it or not, there are lots of those in the market! Just make sure to stock up on any of these: avocado, blackberries, raspberries, strawberries, blueberries, lime, lemon, and coconut. Also, note that tomatoes are fruits too, so feel free to make side dishes or dips with loads of tomatoes! Keep in mind that these fruits should be eaten fresh and not out of a can. If you do eat them fresh off the can, however, take a good look at the nutritional information at the back of the packaging. Avocadoes are particularly popular for those practicing the Ketogenic Diet because they contain LOTS of the good kind of fat.

MEAT AND EGGS

While some diets will tell you to skip the meat, the Ketogenic Diet encourages its consumption. Meat is packed with protein that will feed your muscles and give you a consistent source of energy throughout the day. It's a slow but sure burn when you eat protein as opposed to carbohydrates, which are burned faster and therefore stored faster if you don't use them immediately.

But what kind of meat should you be eating? There's chicken, beef, pork, venison, turkey, and lamb. Keep in mind that quality plays a huge role here – you should be eating grass-fed organic beef or organic poultry if you want to make the most out of this food variety. The nuclear option lets you limit the possibility of ingesting toxins in your body due to the production process of these products. Plus, the preservation process also means there are added salt or sugar in the meat, which can throw off the whole diet.

NUTS AND SEEDS

Nuts and seeds you should add in your cart include chia seeds, brazil nuts, macadamia nuts, flaxseed, walnuts, hemp seeds, pecans, sesame seeds, almonds, hazelnut, and pumpkin seeds. They also contain lots of protein and very little sugar, so they're great if you have the munchies. They're the ideal snack because they're quick, easy, and will keep you

149

full. They're high in calories, though, which is why lots of people steer clear of them. As I mentioned earlier, though – the Ketogenic Diet has nothing to do with calories and everything to do with the nutrient you're eating. So don't pay too much attention to the calorie count and just remember that they're a good source of fats and protein.

DAIRY PRODUCTS

OK – some people in their 50s already have a hard time processing dairy products, but for those who don't – you can happily add many of these to your diet. Make sure to consume sufficient amounts of cheese, plain Greek yogurt, cream butter, and cottage cheese. These dairy products are packed with calcium, protein, and a healthy kind of fat.

OILS

Nope, we're not talking about essentials oils but rather MCT oil, coconut oil, avocado oil, nut oils, and even extra-virgin olive oil. You can start using those for your frying needs to create healthier food options. The beauty of these oils is that they add flavor to the food, making sure you don't get bored quickly with the recipes. Try picking up different types of Keto-friendly oils to add some variety to your cooking.

COFFEE AND TEA

The good news is that you don't have to skip coffee if you're going on a Ketogenic Diet. The bad news is that you can't go to Starbucks anymore and order their blended coffee choices. Instead, beverages would be limited to unsweetened tea or unsweetened coffee to keep sugar consumption low. Opt for organic coffee and tea products to make the most out of these powerful antioxidants.

DARK CHOCOLATE

Yes – chocolate is still on the menu, but it is limited to just dark chocolate. Technically, this means eating chocolate that is 70 percent cacao, which would make the taste a bit bitter.

SUGAR SUBSTITUTES

While sweeteners are an important part of food preparation, you can't just use any kind of sugar in your recipe. Remember: the regular sugar is pure carbohydrate. Even if you're not eating carbohydrates, if you're dumping lots of sugar in your food – you're not following the Ketogenic Diet principles.

So what do you do? You find sugar substitutes. The good news is that there are LOTS of those in the market. You can get rid of the old sugar and use any of these as a good substitute.

Stevia: This is perhaps the most familiar one in this list. It's a natural sweetener derived from plants and contains very few calories. Unlike your regular sugar, stevia may help lower the sugar levels instead of causing it to spike. Note, though, that it's sweeter than actual sugar, so when cooking with stevia, you'll need to lower the amount used. Typically, the ratio is 200 grams of sugar per 1 teaspoon of powdered stevia.

Sucralose: It contains zero calories and zero carbohydrates. It's an artificial sweetener and does not metabolize – hence the complete lack of carbohydrates. Splenda is a sweetener derived from sucralose. Note, though, that you don't want to use this as a baking substitute for sugar. Its best use is for coffee, yogurt, and oatmeal sweetening. Note though that like stevia, it's also very sweet, it's actually 600 times sweeter than the regular sugar. Use sparingly.

Erythritol: It's a naturally occurring compound that interacts with the tongue's sweet taste receptors. Hence, it mimics the taste of sugar without actually being sugar. It does contain calories, but only about 5% of the calories you'll find in the regular sugar. Note, though, that it doesn't dissolve very well, so anything prepared with this sweetener will have a gritty feeling. This can be problematic if you're using the product for baking. As for sweetness, the typical ratio is 1 1/3 cup for 1 cup of sugar.

Xylitol: Like erythritol, xylitol is a type of sugar alcohol that's commonly used in sugar-free gum. While it still contains calories, the calories are just 3 per gram. It's a sweetener that's good for diabetic patients because it doesn't raise the sugar levels of insulin in the body. The great thing about this is that you don't have to do any computations when using it for baking, cooking, or fixing a drink. The ratio of it with sugar is 1 to 1, so you can quickly make the substitution in the recipe.

FOODS TO AVOID

BREAD AND GRAINS

Bread is a staple food in many countries. You have loaves, bagels, tortillas, and the list goes on. However, no matter what form bread takes, they still pack a lot of carbs. The same applies to whole-grain as well because they are made from refined flour.

Depending on your daily carb limit, eating a sandwich or bagel can put your way over your daily limit. So if you really want to eat bread, it is best to make keto variants at home instead.

Grains such as rice, wheat, and oats pack a lot of carbs as well. So limit or avoid that as well.

FRUITS

Fruits are healthy for you. In fact, they have been linked to a lower risk of heart disease and cancer. However, there are a few that you need to avoid in your keto diets. The problem is that some of those foods pack quite a lot of carbs such as banana, raisins, dates, mango, and pear.

As a general rule, avoid sweet and dried fruits. Berries are an exception because they do not contain as much sugar and are rich in fiber. So you can still eat some of them, around 50 grams. Moderation is key.

VEGETABLES

Vegetables are just as healthy for your body. Most of the keto diet does not care how many vegetables you eat so long as they are low in starch. Vegetables that are rich in fiber can help with weight loss. For one, they make you feel full for longer so they help suppress your appetite. Another benefit is that your body would burn more calories to break and digest them. Moreover, they help control blood sugar and aid with your bowel movements.

But that also means you need to avoid or limit vegetables that are high in starch because they have more carbs than fiber. That includes corn, potato, sweet potato, and beets.

PASTA

Pasta is also a staple food in many countries. It is versatile and convenient. As with any other convenient food, pasta is rich in carbs. So when you are on your keto diet, spaghetti or any other types of pasta are not recommended. You can probably get away with it by eating a small portion, but that is not possible.

Thankfully, that does not mean you need to give up on it altogether. If you are craving pasta, you can try some other alternatives that are low in carbs such as spiralized veggies or shirataki noodles.

CEREAL

Cereal is also a huge offender because sugary breakfast cereals pack a lot of carbs. That also applies to "healthy cereals." Just because they use other words to describe their product does not mean that you should believe them. That also applies to oatmeal, whole-grain cereals, etc.

So when you eat a bowl of cereal when you are doing keto, you are already way over your carb limit, and we haven't even added milk into the equation! Therefore, avoid whole-grain cereal or cereals that we mention here altogether.

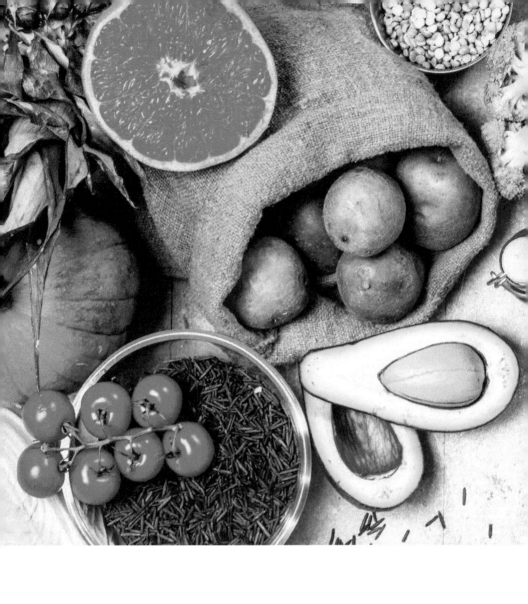

CHAPTER 04

HOW DOES AGIN AFFECT YOUR NUTRITIONAL NEEDS

Chapter 04 - How Does Aging Affect Your Nutritional Needs

Nutrition is vital to maintain health and to lead an active and fulfilling life. There is another fact that your nutritional need changes throughout your life and that's why eating healthy becomes more important. If you are eating unhealthy food and suffering from nutritional deficiencies, then this will bring harmful outcomes, and you will lead a poor quality life.

Childhood: In the initial years of life, the little bodies need essential nutrients along with natural nutrients to ensure they develop and grow physically and mentally. The food should provide high energy to support the rapid growth of bodies at this age. Also, childhood is the time of learning and experiencing new foods and developing taste and smell sense, which shape their eating habits for later in life. Therefore, children should be encouraged to consume a variety of foods every day.

The key nutrient in children diet includes protein which is necessary for growth, calcium, and vitamin D to grow strong bones.

Along with these nutrients, vitamin A is also crucial for developing a healthy immune system, and zinc and iron make the children mentally fit and ready for all the learning experiences at their school.

Adolescence: The body around this time goes through significant emotional and physical changes due to puberty. Moreover, maturing sexuality increases muscle growth and strengthens the bones, and this is a perfect opportunity for children to build strong bones for later. For this reason, the body must meet its calcium requirement. For this, dairy milk products are perfect healthy choices such as yogurt, milk, and cheese that are well known for high-quality protein and calcium-rich sources. Iron is also an essential bone nutrient that can be obtained from red meat, chicken, kidney beans, spinach, and mussels.

Teenage is also a time when children often tend to opt for junk foods and sugary drinks over more nutritious options. Encourage them to have water or milk as beverages and healthy snacks to combat craving and untimely hunger. Also, make-ahead some smoothies, prepare grab-and-go food options like toasts and sandwiches, and do meal prep for children that can't sit long enough to eat food at the meal table.

Adulthood: This is the time when you have to focus on maintaining the healthy body you have developed through your childhood and adolescence. Therefore, the body should get good enough nutrition like protein, calcium, vitamins, and phosphorus that helps you stay active, energetic, and maintain bones and muscles that tend to decrease as we move forward in age. Focus on eating healthy foods that give you all the nutrients, which make you feel great without disturbing your ideal body weight and reduce the factors of ailments like diabetes and heart diseases.

Older age: At the old age, the body needs the same or even more protein, minerals, and vitamins. For example, after the age of 50, your body's ability to absorb specific vitamins fades due to hormonal changes, and you don't have enough stomach acid to break down food sources. So, if you aren't eating foods that don't have these vitamins or not taking nutrients supplements, then you may suffer from dangerous ailments. In that case, eat little and often can effectively help your body in getting essential nutrients that support mobility, active mind, growth, mental and physical performance. Enjoy a variety of foods and drinks and go for nutritious and natural options for foods that contain a range of nutrients. Similarly, you may not notice thirst in your later years, but keeping your body hydrated is important at any age.

With these examples, you have to make little bits of changes in what you eat and drink to achieve optimal health no matter what your age is.

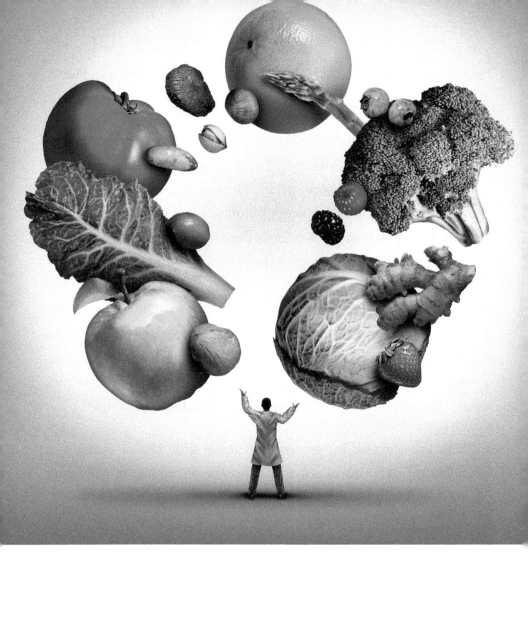

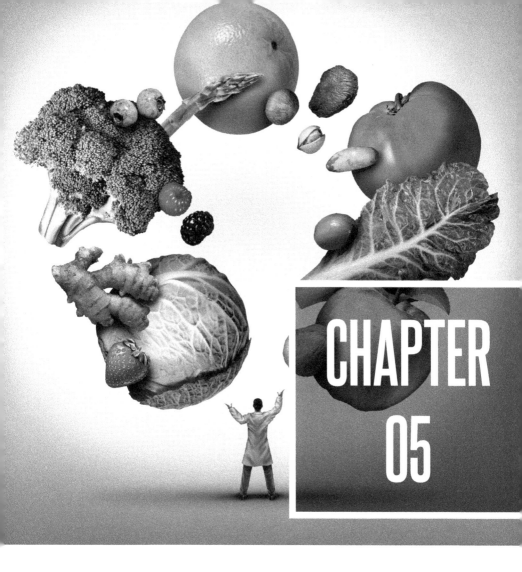

CHAPTER 05

THE SCIENCE BEHIND
THE KETO DIET

Chapter 05 - The Science Behind the Keto Diet

To bring the body into a ketogenic condition, you need to follow a high-fat diet and small carbohydrates without any grains, or almost any. The composition will be roughly 80% fat and 20% protein. For the very first two days, that will be the rule.

You need to eat a high-fat diet and minimal carbs without any grains, or almost any, to bring the body into a ketogenic condition. The composition would be about 80% fat and 20% protein. This will be the law for the very first two days.

When the body absorbs carbs, it induces an insulin surge that has the insulin emitted by the pancreas, and common sense assures us that if we then eliminate carbs, the insulin does not hold excess calories as the perfect fat. The body today has no carbs as an energy source, so your body should look for a new source.

If you decide to remove extra weight, this works well. The body must break down the extra fat and function with it, rather than carbs, as energy.

That particular condition is known as Ketosis. This state in which you want the body to be in, can make great sense in case you want to drop excess fat while keeping muscle.

Let's move on now to the portion of the diet, and how to prepare it. With every pound of lean mass, you would need to ingest no less than one gram of protein. It will aid with strengthening and restoring muscle tissue during exercises. That means 65% protein and 30% fat.

Effectively if you weigh 150 pounds, that means 150 g of protein a day. If you multiply it four times (number of calories equivalent to 600 calories in a gram of protein), any of the calories will come from fat. If the caloric maintenance is 3000, you need to consume about 500, less that might imply that one day if you require 2500 calories, about 1900 calories should come from the fats!

To fuel the body, you have to consume fats, which in exchange will also burn up excess fat! That is the diet plan rule; you've got to consume fats! The downside of taking healthy fats and the keto diet is that you're not going to be thirsty. Fat processing of food is slow, operating to the benefit and making you feel whole.

You're going to be working on Monday-Friday, and then on the other days, you're going to have a 'carb-up.' When this process begins when the last exercise is on Friday, post-training, you need to take a liquid carbohydrate with your whey shake. This will help produce an insulin surge, which also allows us to provide the carbohydrates that the body urgently requires for restoring muscle mass and for glycogen stores to expand & refill.

Consume whatever you like during this specific process (carb up)- pizzas, crisps, spaghetti, ice cream. Somehow, this will be beneficial for you because it can refresh the body for the week ahead and provide the food that your body requires.

Switch your focus onto the no-carb high-fat average protein diet program as Sunday starts. Holding the body in Ketosis and losing fat is the optimal remedy, by muscle.

An additional benefit of Ketosis is when you enter the ketosis state and burn the fat, the body will deplete from carbohydrates. Packing up with carbs can make you appear as full as before (but even fewer body fat!), perfect for holiday activities if you visit the seaside or parties!

Let us recap on the diet schedule today.

Get in ketosis state by removing carbs and taking moderate/low protein, high fat.

Take some kind of fiber to keep the pipes as clear as ever, should you realize what I mean.

If the ketosis protein consumption has been collected, per pound of lean mass will be no less than that of a g of protein.

So it is! It does require determination not to eat carbs during the week because certain products contain carbs; however, note that you would be greatly rewarded for the devotion.

You must not live on end days in the condition of Ketosis, because it is dangerous and will wind up with yourself turning to make use of protein as a source of food that is a no-no.

Ketogenic diet systems are structured primarily to trigger a ketosis condition within the body. If the volume of glucose within the body is low, the whole body turns to fat as a source of energy replacement.

The body has main sources of fuel, one of which is:

GLUCOSE

Free fatty acids (FFA) and, to a lesser degree, ketones from FFA Fat by-products are kept in the triglyceride type. Typically, they are split into long-chain fatty acids and glycerol.

The removal of glycerol from the triglyceride molecule enables the three free fatty acid (FFA) molecules to be used as energy for the introduction into the bloodstream.

The molecule of glycerol goes into the liver, where three molecules of it combine to create one molecule of sugar. Additionally, when the body consumes fat, it creates glucose as a by-product. Its glucose may be used to power different regions of the brain and body parts that can't operate on FFA molecules.

However, though glucose on its triglycerides will travel through the blood, cholesterol takes a carrier to go through the bloodstream. In a carrier known as LDL or low-density lipoprotein, cholesterol and triglycerides are packed. Thus, the larger the LDL particles, the greater the number of triglycerides it has.

The general process of energy-burning of fat deposits produces co2, oxygen, and ketone-known components. The liver produces ketones out of the free essential fatty acids. Right now, they consist of two classes of atoms jointly joined by a purposeful carbonyl unit.

The body cannot shop ketones, and therefore they should be used or excreted at times. The body often excretes them as acetone through the breath, and as acetoacetate through the urine.

The ketones may be used as a source of energy for body cells. The subconscious will use ketones to generate between 70-75 percent of the energy requirement.

As for alcoholic drinks, ketones take priority over carbohydrates as food resources. That means that they should be consumed first when filled with the bloodstream before glucose can be used as a fuel.

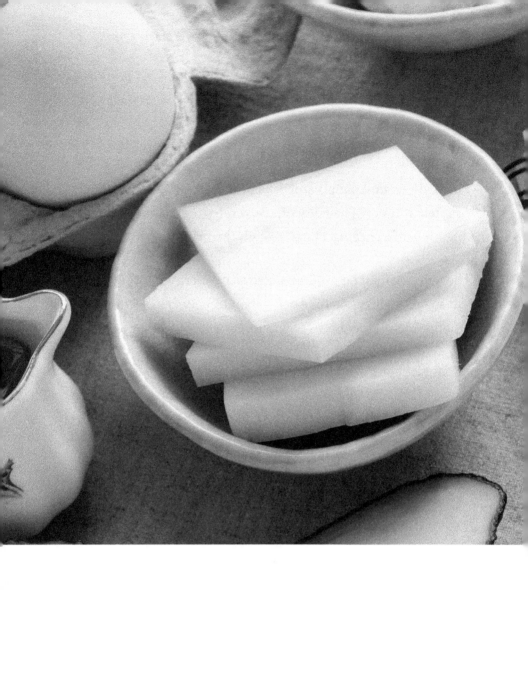

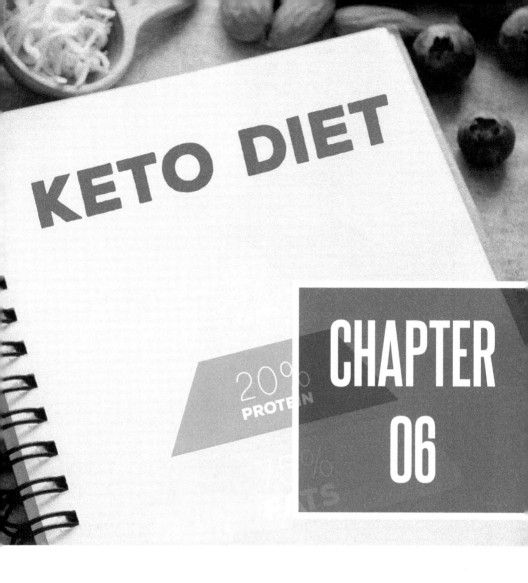

THE TOP 12 KETO
MYTHS DEBUNKED

Caphter 06 - The Top 12 Keto Myths Debunked

Myths and misconceptions are simply false or wrong ideas or concepts that people tend to have and use them. If you have decided to give the Ketogenic diet a go, these myths and misconceptions could make the whole process a challenge or increase the chance that you will not attempt the diet or even lead you to health risks if you opted to believe them. It is important to note that approaching the decision to try the diet with adequate knowledge on all the positives, negatives as well as myths and misconceptions could set you up for success.

Take a look at these myths and misconceptions prepared for you:

The Keto diet allows you to eat as much butter as you want: even though the Ketogenic diet is a diet that is rich in fats, it does not mean that you could eat as much butter as you would prefer. It is very easy to convince yourself that you are doing the right thing, but realizing that the diet does not allow you to eat all sorts of fats is very important.

The healthiest way to regulate your fat consumption is by limiting your consumption of saturated fats and improving on your intake of unsaturated fats such as olive oil or avocados but in moderation. This myth could mislead you into overfeeding on fats and risk other complications as a result of too many fats.

Reality: The Ketogenic diet advocates for the consumption of unsaturated fats in your diet rather than just any fats.

You could go on or off the Ketogenic diet and still lose weight: out of curiosity, most people would adopt the diet with the hope of shedding off extra weight but without consulting with their physicians or doctors. As a result, they could end up starting the Ketogenic diet for one day and regularly switch to the regular diet and still expect to shed off the extra weight. For you to achieve and maintain the state of Ketosis, you would be required to stick solely to the Ketogenic diet. This is because switching to the regular diet removes your body from Ketosis, and your body goes back to burning carbohydrates instead of fats, thus shedding that extra weight becomes a problem. The only way you are going to benefit from the diet is if you strictly maintain your eating habits in line with the diet

Reality: Shifting your attention away from the diet could lead you to gain more weight rather than shed it.

The Ketogenic diet is the best for weight loss: just because someone you know started and benefitted from the diet does not mean the diet would do the same for you, just because a friend of yours lost weight while on a diet does not guarantee that the diet could do the same for you. Or perhaps, given the fact that everyone around you is trying the diet does not mean that you should try it as well. You should be in a position to know that the only way you could shed off that extra weight is that you are consistent. It is after this that you could decide to adopt the diet and not simply because everyone around you is trying it. You should be in a position to know that there are other ways to lose weight as well as other diets to do the same. Keep an open mind and pick on a way or a diet that would best suit all your needs.

Reality: Other diets could be used to shed weight as well as other ways to shed weight.

One person's Ketogenic diet meal plan could work for everyone: it is very easy to assume that another person's Ketogenic meal plan could also work for you. You should be able to understand that another person's body needs and requirements are different to your body's needs and requirements. Their intake of carbohydrates is very different from yours, and so are their dietary needs different from yours. This is why it is not advisable to jump into someone else's Ketogenic diet. However, instead, it is wise to visit your doctor or physician or nutritionist to get your own dietary needs evaluated and properly met in your meal plan.

Reality: Someone else's Ketogenic meal plan is unique only to them, and getting your own Ketogenic meal plan is wise.

Going into Ketosis is equal to going into ketoacidosis: Ketosis is a state in which the body learns to burn fats rather than the preferred carbohydrates for energy. During Ketosis, your body converts fats into ketone bodies, which take the place of glucose from carbohydrates and become your body's energy. Confusing Ketosis with ketoacidosis, which is a life-threatening complication resulting from diabetes, could be very lethal. This is because you could relax and assume that just because you adopted the Ketogenic diet that your body is in Ketosis. It is advisable to visit your doctor if you feel adverse changes to your body rather than assuming other things.

Reality: You could lose your life simply by ignoring changes to your body and making your diagnosis. Administering self-treatment could be fatal.

You cannot eat fruits while on the Keto diet: it is true that fruits and vegetables are great sources of carbohydrates and that the only things that could be free from carbohydrates are oils or meat. It is easy to believe that you should not eat fruits while on the Ketogenic diet, but the truth is that some fruits and vegetables are Keto-friendly. Fruits such as berries are low in carbs, and that makes them Keto-friendly, as well as zucchini and broccoli, which are low carb vegetables that you could ingest. This is why it is important to visit your doctor or nutritionist to get your meal plan in line and one which will cater to all your needs.

Reality: You need to consult with your physician before ruling out foods on a diet.

You Don't Need a Good Plan

Reality: You must have a well-formulated plan.

Many studies have indicated this is where the dieters go wrong on the concept of losing weight quickly. A well-formulated ketogenic diet will consist of moderate protein and low carbs. That's where many studies cited by critics seem to get it wrong. Sometimes, it is merely where you have incorrectly calculated your macros. Or, you might make an error when calculating the net carbs. To reach net carbs, which is the number you use to calculate your daily carbohydrates, you take the total amount of carbs minus the fiber counts to come up with net carbs. A well-formulated ketogenic diet will have the majority of fats based on saturated fats.

You don't need time to adapt to the plan

Reality: You have to realize the adaption time of the ketogenic diet plan can take anywhere from two to four weeks or more. For some, it can take as much as six to eight weeks. It takes time because you cannot instantly switch over to using fat as a fuel source. It takes time for your body to adjust to the changes. You may be experiencing low energy, withdrawal-type symptoms, fatigue, or headaches, but they will pass.

Your Brain Needs Sugar/Glucose

Reality: Your body doesn't need sugar to function properly. This is true only if your body is in a sugar-burning mode. Using a well-structured ketogenic adapted diet, your brain runs on ketones. There's still some glucose required, but it can be easily supplied by protein. Protein is your preferred fuel source for the brain. You will also see improvements in mental acuity, cognition, moods, focus, and so much more using the keto plan.

You should not use the Keto plan for extended periods

Reality: Most of the misconception about the diet plan over the short-term is perceived as health risks of the ketogenic diet. The ketogenic plan is a lifestyle change. It leads to improvement in both short and long-term health. As noted, the keto lifestyle is excellent for losing weight and reversing autoimmune issues. In the long term, it can help stave off cancer, diabetes, Alzheimer's, coronary artery disease, and so much more. How can it not be useful in the long term?

The keto diet can inhibit growth in kids

Reality: This is one of the concepts that is not true. Many of the studies cited have been conducted on children with cerebral palsy and epilepsy. It's a well-known fact that both of these health issues can cause growth problems. Since these children are in a category that has problems with growth, it is merely stated by some that the keto diet is the cause of inhibited growth in kids. Very untrue!

The keto diet can put me into ketoacidosis

Reality: Ketosis is what causes you to burn fat on the keto diet. During the process, your body's breaking down the fat into ketone bodies. According to the Mayo Clinic, this is a different thing as a diabetic ketoacidosis incident, which is a potentially life-threatening complication of diabetes that can happen when your body doesn't get enough insulin and ketone levels are high at the same time.

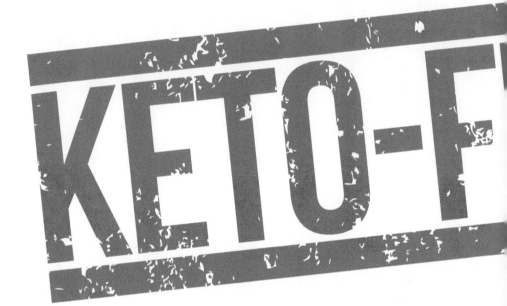

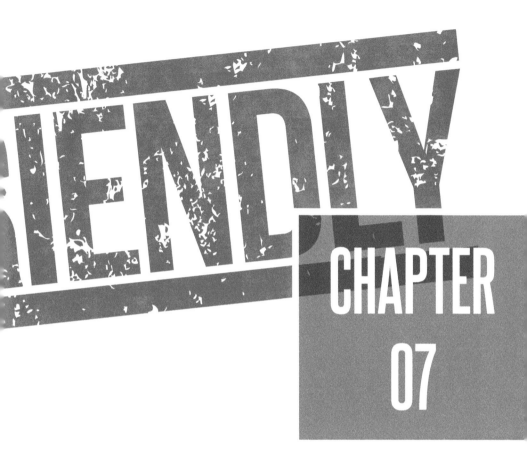

CHAPTER 07

THE WORST SIDE EFFECTS OF THE KETO DIET

Chapter 07 - The Worst Side Effects of the Keto Diet

KETO BREATH

One of the most common side effects of a keto diet is bad breath. Not everyone who adopts the keto diet experiences this problem, but it is common. Bad breath comes as a result of internal metabolism processes. Your liver metabolizes the massive amounts of fat you are consuming and then converts them to ketone bodies such as the acetone. These ketone bodies are broken down into smaller organizations and are then circulated inside your body. As the ketone bodies circulate, it gets into your lungs through the diffusion process, and eventually, it is exerted out through your breath.

HOW TO OVERCOME KETO BREATH

You can control bad keto breath by increasing water intake. You can also get rid of this problem by practicing good oral hygiene like regularly brushing your teeth. Alternatively, you can mask ketosis odor using mints and gums. It is also advisable to eat slightly more carbs and less protein if you have this problem.

KETO FLU

You may experience symptoms resembling those of flu, especially during your first days on a keto diet. Such symptoms include aches, fatigue, cramping, skin rash, and diarrhea. The side effects are caused by dehydration as a result of your body losing a lot of water and electrolytes.

When your body uses fat to fuel its functions instead of using protein, you tend to lose more water and electrolytes through urination. The loss of water and electrolytes is accelerated further by the low insulin levels and muscle glycogen that accompanies the keto diet.

Besides, most keto diets consist of food with little water and potassium levels, further accelerating the loss of body water and electrolytes.

HOW TO OVERCOME KETO FLU

You can handle keto flu by drinking a lot of water. You can also eat lots of soup. If you get enough rest, you will give your body enough energy to fight the flu on its own.

You need to lower the effects of keto flu by getting enough sleep. You can also drink a lot of water to minimize the impact of keto flu. There are also some supplements found in natural sources like organic coffee or matcha tea that could help you overcome the flu. Make a point to get enough salts and electrolytes, too.

FATIGUE

You may experience extreme feelings of tiredness once you adopt a keto diet. Fatigue is caused by a lack of glucose reaching your brain. Although this side effect will last for a few days, it could still cause much discomfort and worry on your part.

HOW TO OVERCOME KETO FATIGUE

Drink a lot of water and get enough rest. You can also avoid engaging in strenuous exercises. You can also eat healthy carbs to give you the extra energy your body needs.

GI SIDE EFFECTS

Keto diet can also harm your digestive system over the long term. Keto diet has been thought to cause some stomach problems such as constipation high cholesterol levels, diarrhea, kidneys stones, and vomiting.

You may also experience abnormal stomach gas due to the sugar alcohols found in some keto diets, for example, the sugars found in some processed foods. The higher the amount of food you eat, the higher the impact of the side effects on you.

How to control GI problems when you are on a keto diet

Drink lots of water and eat high fiber foods such as fruits and vegetables to encourage the growth of beneficial bacteria in your GI system. Make it a habit of exercising regularly.

Weakened immune system

Keto diets can also weaken the immune systems of some people. Studies suggest that keto foods could cause a condition called dysbiosis. Dysbiosis occurs when the balance of helpful and harmful bacteria is altered in your GI tract. The disruption is caused by the consumption of highly saturated fats and low fiber levels in your digestive system.

When you ingest diets with little prebiotic fiber, the number of beneficial bacteria decreases substantially in your digestive system. Your GI tract is the backbone of your immune system, and any compromise to it could have a negative impact on the immune functions leading to exposure to chronic diseases.

How to avoid weakened immune system when on a keto diet

Incorporate workouts to your keto diet. You can also eat high fiber food, such as fruits and vegetables. Also, ensure you drink lots of water.

VITAMIN AND OTHER MINERAL DEFICIENCIES

If you are on the keto diet, you may not receive enough vitamins and minerals needed for your body to function normally. Plant-based minerals such as calcium and vitamin D may not be present in your keto diet in the quantities required by your body. If these minerals decrease in your body for long periods, you may stand a high risk of getting lifestyle diseases such as heart failure.

The heart failure comes as a result of the hardening of your heart muscles because of the lack of enough selenium. Selenium is an essential immune-boosting antioxidant usually occurring in plant-based food. Lack of this critical antioxidant causes the hardening of your heart muscles leading to heart failure.

How to treat the deficiencies when you are on a keto diet

Eat lots of fruits and vegetables to get vitamins. You can also use beneficial supplements to treat any deficiencies, which comes with the keto diet.

INCREASED RISK OF CHRONIC DISEASE

The Keto diet requires you to put a limit on the number of carbohydrates and protein you consume. When you eat much fat to get enough calories needed by your body, you will be limiting fiber-rich foods such as vegetables, fruits, or legumes. These foods are some of the best sources of immune-boosting nutrients needs by your body to stay healthy. Therefore, when you limit these nutrients in your body, you increase your risk of getting chronic diseases such as diabetes, cancer, high blood pressure.

Studies show that diets that are high in fruits and vegetables can significantly reduce chronic diseases. The more you consume them, the better you are health-wise. When you restrict their consumption, you tend to decrease their beneficial impacts.

How to reduce the risk of chronic diseases when on keto diets

We'll say it again: drink lots of water. Eat lots of fruits and vegetables. You can also incorporate exercise into your keto diet to get the best results.

Chronic inflammation

Studies show that when you consume high fats needed for Ketosis, your cholesterol and lipoprotein structure could be significantly altered and will result in inflammation over a while. Inflammation occurs when the cells of your body use much energy to accomplish their normal functioning. Chronic inflammation is also one of the causes of heart diseases.

How to minimize chronic inflammation when on keto diets

You can control the problem of inflammation by eating solid fats and oils. Ensure you also include high fiber foods in your daily intake, like fruits and vegetables.

THE CHALLENGE OF WEIGHT CYCLING

When you restrict your eating diets for an extended period, you may end up gaining too much weight when not dieting, which you then go ahead and lose when on a diet. This process of alternating between weight gain and weight loss is what is referred to as weight cycling. Weight cycling can increase the risk of getting chronic diseases.

HOW TO CONTROL WEIGHT CYCLING

You can control weight cycling by shortening the intervals between dieting and the days you are on free diets. You should gradually increase the amount of food you consume during your free diet days so that your body can have enough time to adjust to the changes in your program.

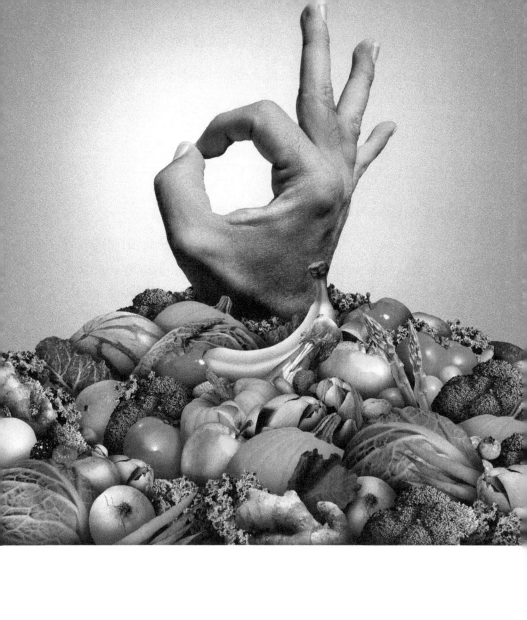

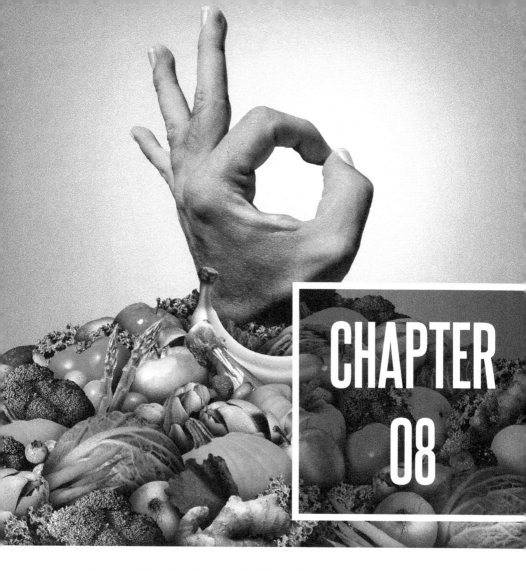

CHAPTER 08

THE IMPORTANCE OF THE EXERCISING FOR SENIORS BENEFITS AND MYTHS

Chapter 08 - The Importance of Exercising for Seniors Benefits and Myths

Exercising offers a plethora of benefits to all, regardless of your age! Healthy movement results in improved flexibility and stronger bones, which is quite important for older folks. You see, as you age, your body's muscle mass starts to decrease. As we enter our forties, adults begin to lose three to five percent of muscle mass as they enter each new decade.

However, we do realize how the thought of exercising regularly at an older age can seem like a challenge, especially if you're feeling let down with frequent aches and pains. But in many ways, the benefits of exercising outweigh the potential risks. Let's dive into why exercising is such important for seniors.

BENEFITS AND MYTHS OF EXERCISING FOR SENIORS

Now, while you may be having thoughts about exercising, here are a couple of benefits that you can't ignore:

• Prevents Diseases

Regular physical activity has been known to reduce the risks of diseases such as diabetes and heart disease. This is mainly because exercise strengthens overall immune functioning, which is particularly beneficial for seniors who are often immunocompromised. So even if you can't hit the gym, some form of light exercise can play an integral role in disease management.

• Helps Increase Social Ties and Prevents Isolation

Aging can be a daunting process, but it becomes fun when a community surrounds you. Opting for yoga or fitness classes not only makes exercising more fun, but it also helps you strengthen social ties with other older adults in your neighborhood. This can help ward off the occasional loneliness that one is likely to feel at old age. Plus, this will help you stay committed to your goals and lead a healthier lifestyle.

• Improves Cognitive Function

Regular exercise can also improve fine motor skills that boost cognitive function. Several studies have shown how exercising regularly can reduce the risk of dementia.

Unfortunately, older folks have a higher risk of falling, which can lead to serious injuries. This can also drastically reduce your chances of leading an independent life as you grow older. As seniors take much longer to recover from injuries and falls, it is important to exercise to improve balance add mobility.

Myths on Exercising

There are some myths associated with exercising for seniors. Let's debunk those misconceptions today:

Myth 1: I'm going to grow older, what's the point of exercising

Now, you might be thinking, "why should I exercise when moving around is likely to get difficult as I grow older?" Now here's the thing physical activity improves balance and helps you stay independent much longer. If you start exercising in your fifties, you are likely to have a better time moving around in your seventies, so start now.

Myth 2: I won't be great at exercising because I'm old

First off, you're never too old to exercise! So while strength and muscle mass tend to decline with age, that doesn't mean you can't partake in any form of physical activity. It's time you set healthier goals for yourself and improve your health. After all, isn't what this keto journey's all about? The key to exercising is finding activities that are suitable for you.

Living a sedentary lifestyle won't do you any good and will take a toll on your body.

MYTH 3: I'LL BE AT A GREATER RISK OF FALLING DOWN

If you're not careful, you will fall regardless of your age. Regular physical activity builds stamina and strength. In many ways, exercising can help improve balance, reducing the risks of falling.

MYTH 4: I'M NOT ATHLETIC, I PROBABLY AM NOT FIT ENOUGH TO EXERCISE

Here's some news for you: our bodies are quite adjustable. So if you've suddenly decided to live a healthier lifestyle, nothing should stop you. So even if you're not athletic, that's perfectly fine, your body can still adjust to your new routine. Start with gentle activities such as brisk walking and then start building up from there.

MYTH 5: I HAVE A DISABILITY AND CAN'T EXERCISE

People who are specially-abled or are chair-bound may find exercising challenging, but that doesn't mean you can't be part of the fan. Take up chair yoga or lift light weights. Tons of simple exercises can help you improve the range of motion and flexibility. Speak to your doctor and, hopefully, should have some great tips for you to follow.

Simple Exercises for Seniors

Here is a list of simple exercises that people in their fifties and beyond can enjoy:

Light Weight Training

You can start with a little weight training to retain bone density and build muscle mass. If you're more interested in doing home exercises than joining the gym, invest in 2-pound weights, and perform arm raises and shoulder presses.

Ideally, we recommend that you join a fitness center or gym where you can meet like-minded folks. You can also get yourself a personal trainer who can recommend customized workouts for you. Either way, remember to take it slow at first as you don't want to exert yourself too much.

Walking

If lifting weights isn't for you, good old-fashioned walking should also work for you. Consider taking a nice walk around your neighborhood or go to a park nearby. You'll be able to make some friends and enjoy the weather while you're at it too.

In case you'd rather workout at home, strap on a pedometer, and get going around the house. You'll be able to get more out of this workout if you move your arms and lift your knees as you take each step.

AEROBICS

Joining an aerobics class can significantly help you keep your muscles strong while maintaining mobility. This will not only improve balance but will reduce the risk of falls, thus drastically improving the overall quality of your life as you grow older.

Many studies have also indicated how aerobic exercises can protect memory and sharpen your mind and improving cognitive function among older adults. If you're not comfortable joining a class, you'll find plenty of videos online. Aerobic exercises have also been known to get the heart pumping, improving cardiovascular help.

SWIMMING

Do you find regular exercise too boring? Swimming is a fun, impact-free exercise that can get you through the day. It's almost pain-free and won't trouble your aging joints. Swimming offers resistance training and will help you get back up to your feet again.

Here's how it works: the water offers gentle resistance while giving you a cardiovascular workout too. This also builds muscle capacity and helps you build strength too.

YOGA

What's not to love about yoga? It's relaxing, it's healthy, and you can enjoy it with a group. Yoga does an excellent job of improving flexibility in your joints. It allows seniors to remain limber and maintain their sense of balance. If you have trouble moving about or stretching, then you can try chair yoga.

Some classic yoga poses that you might want to try out include seated forward bend, downward-facing dog, and warrior.

SQUATS

When you're working on an exercise program, you shouldn't skip the idea of strength training. Squats happen to be an excellent way to strengthen the muscles of your lower body. Doing squats is relatively easy, and you won't need any sort of equipment except for maybe a chair to support yourself. However, if you have trouble with balance, we suggest you skip this exercise and opt for something much simpler.

SIT-UPS

Sit-ups are a great way to strengthen your core muscles, improve back pain problems, and balance. Performing simple sit-ups should do the job. All you have to do is lie down on your back and keep your knees bent at an angle. Now place your hands behind your head and then gently try to lift your head. You should feel the sensation in your core muscles.

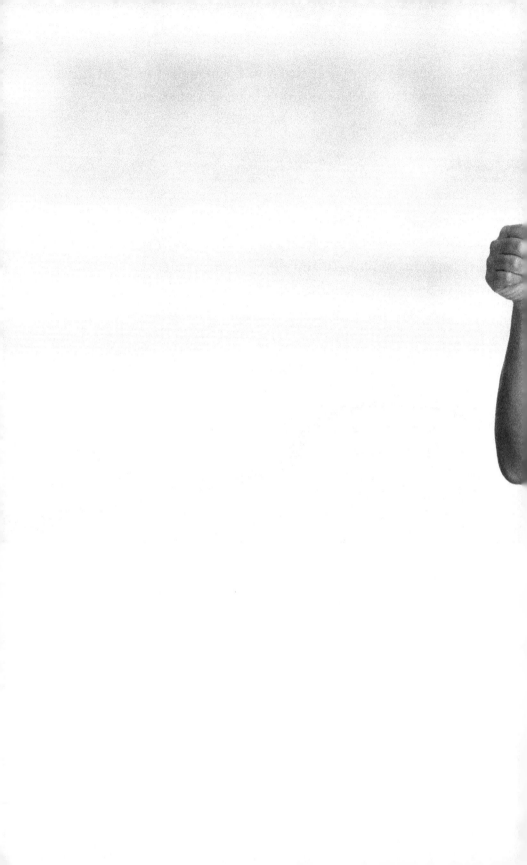

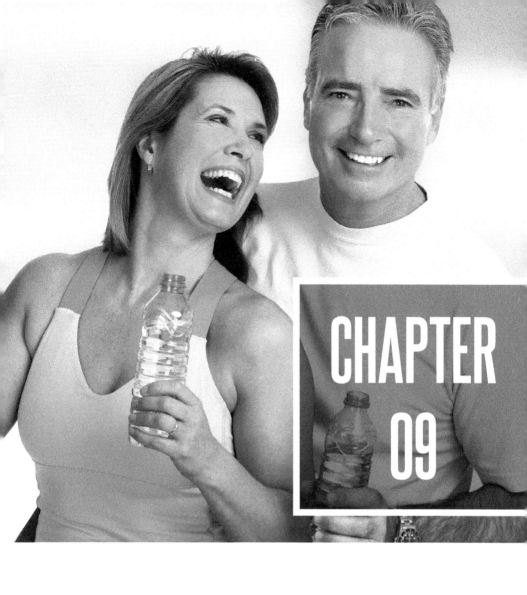

CHAPTER

09

EXERCISES TO ASSIST WITH QUALITY OF LIFE AFTER 50

Chapter 09 - Exercises to Assist with Quality of Life After 50

Age really is just a number. You might be 55, but look 40 and feel 35. Or, you might be 50, but look and feel 65. It all has to do with how well you care for your body and what you do to stay active.

When it comes to exercise, many people assume if they weren't active during their 20s, 30s or 40s, there's no point in getting started in their 50s or even later. Fortunately, that's just not true. It's never too late to start an exercise program. Starting a workout routine can help reverse some of the problems caused by inactivity and can make you feel great about yourself overall.

Let's take a closer look at the benefits of exercise for women over the age of 50 and at some of the different types of exercises that will help you feel your best.

Muscles in Motion

Set to music from the 1950s and '60s, Muscles in Motion helps you tighten and tone your upper and lower body, with a particular focus on the abdominal muscles. The group class uses hand weights, resistance bands and exercise balls to build strength.

How to Tighten Your Buttocks with Resistance Bands

Just like lifting a heavier weight, adding resistance to a lower body exercise makes it more intense. If you want a truly effective buttock workout, add resistance bands to your donkey kicks and leg lifts. You'll be seeing results in no time.

Lose Weight with the Walk Fast/Slow Plan

This plan will ease you into running. It's a step-by-step guide that is perfect for anyone who is new to running, or people getting back into it after an injury or extended absence. For many women, walking, jogging or running is all the cardio they need to stay healthy.

Plank Pose

The plank not only helps to strengthen and tone your core muscles — also known as your abdominal and lower back muscles — it can improve your balance too. Planks can also help straighten your posture, which is a plus if you sit in a chair for much of the day.

There are several ways to do a plank. For a high plank, get into a position as if you are at the top of a push-up, with your arms and legs straight.

Another option is a low plank, which can be easier to do if you're a beginner. Instead of supporting yourself on your hands, bend your arms at the elbow and support your weight on your forearms.

No matter which version you choose, keep your back completely straight and your head up. Your entire body should form a straight line parallel to the ground.

ON-THE-MAT SIX PACK WORKOUT

This is a basic mat workout you can do anywhere and anytime. You'll notice your abs burning after the first few moves. The trick to getting visible results is to keep your core engaged throughout the workout. Focus on keeping proper form and contracting the abdominal muscles.

6-MINUTE ARM TONING WORKOUT

This dumbbell arm workout will teach you all the basic lifting exercises you need to tone your arms. It will target your biceps, triceps, shoulders, and a little bit of your upper back. Beginners can start with a single round and slowly work their way up from there.

SQUATS WITH A CHAIR

Another weight-burning exercise that's easy to do at home is squats with a chair. During this exercise, you squat over a chair as if you were about to sit down, but don't make contact with the seat. Instead, you stand back up and repeat the process multiple times.

Squats not only help tone your lower body, but they can also help improve balance. When you get started, you might find it's easiest to perform the exercise with your hands and arms extended out in front of you.

CHEST FLY

Women tend to have very weak and underdeveloped chest muscles. The chest fly is a weightlifting exercise that helps strengthen those muscles.

To do the exercise, you'll need a pair of hand weights. Lie on the floor or a mat, flat on your back, with your knees bent and your feet flat on the ground. Take one weight in each hand and raise your arms over your chest.

Slowly, open your arms out to the side, lowering your arms and wrists toward the floor — but don't actually touch the ground. Keep a slight bend in your elbows, so you don't lock out your arms. Raise your arms back up and repeat.

BEFORE BREAKFAST MINI MORNING WORKOUT

A morning workout is more energizing than a cup of coffee. Not to mention cheaper too! This 6-minute workout combines yoga with some basic bodyweight moves to wake you gently. It'll help you stretch, get your blood flowing, and even rev up your mind.

S.O.S.

If you are particularly concerned about the risk of osteoporosis or are concerned about bone loss, S.O.S. is the fitness class for you. It focuses on resistance exercises that help improve bone health and muscle mass.

SilverSneakers Classic

SilverSneakers exercise programs are available free of charge to people on Medicare. The classic program focuses on strength training as well as aerobic activities. Designed for all fitness levels, there are modifications available for people who need additional support or assistance.

Summer Slim Down Workout for Beginners

It's cardio without the treadmill. However, if you push through this workout at a quick pace, you'll burn more calories than you would have running! Squats, walking lunges, hip twists, toe touches, and planks, all activate large muscle groups that help you burn tons of calories. Do this workout 2 to 3 times per week to up your calorie burn.

30-Minute Upper Body Cardio Workout

This 30-minute routine is a complete workout. If you do this, you don't have to do anything else for the day, other than a quick warm-up and cool-down. This workout is more advanced than some of the others on this list, so it's ideal for women who are already fit.

3 Moves to Toned Inner Thighs

This quick 3-move workout is a combination of cardio and lower body strength training. While the moves will challenge your muscles, therefore making them grow stronger, the kicking and stepping also raises your heart rate. You'll be burning calories even while you build muscle.

10-Minute Beginner's Yoga Workout for Balance

One mistake women in their 50s often make is assuming they'll never be able to complete a workout if they don't get through it their first time. The point of this yoga workout is to slowly improve your balance and flexibility. You may struggle with the poses at first! Be persistent and you'll love the results.

The main issue with exercise and keto is that at first, your body enters a transition period where you might experience low energy levels and brain "fog." Deprived of glucose, your body has to adjust to making and using ketone bodies for energy. For some people, this is not a problem, while others will have to adjust to the "keto flu." The good news is that this will pass once your body becomes fully adjusted, and your energy levels will increase.

If you suffer from this issue, you shouldn't stop exercising, but you probably won't want to hit it hard or add new challenges to your exercise routine, either. The key to exercise and keto is consuming enough fat.

Once you transition to keto, fat is your energy source, so it's important that you genuinely consume the levels of fat the diet demands. If you eat enough fat, then you'll have enough energy for your workouts and find that you burn more fat off your body when you do exercise.

Some recent research into the benefits of exercise has uncovered surprises that might be to the liking of most readers. A person had to engage in 20 or 30 minutes of "vigorous" exercise per day to get the benefits. When researchers studied people who were regular runners, however, they came across a stunning result – people who only ran five minutes a day got most of the health benefits that those running 30 minutes or an hour got from their running. The runners were followed over a long period, and it was found that all runners had a lower risk of death and cardiovascular disease as compared to people who didn't exercise, or did so at moderate levels. But the differences between those who ran only five minutes and those running for long periods wasn't all that significant. You can find a nice lay person's discussion of this research in the New York Times.

So, it appears that people get the majority of the benefit that hard cardiovascular training provides after only a short period of exercising.

This surprising result provides an alternative for people who aren't very excited about putting in long days at the gym. It may be possible that you can get the same benefits by just going on a short jog.

Now we aren't giving out specific health advice in this guidebook, so it's up to each individual to do the research and find out what works best for him or her. One possible way to rev up your exercise without having to kill yourself is to do a 30-minute walk three or four days a week, and do a five-minute jog three days a week. That way, you're getting a little bit of both.

At the time of writing, researchers aren't sure if the five-minute benefits accrue to other types of exercise. So they aren't sure if riding on an exercise bike for five minutes a day will provide the same benefits or not, but common sense seems to imply that it would if you use a good level of intensity.

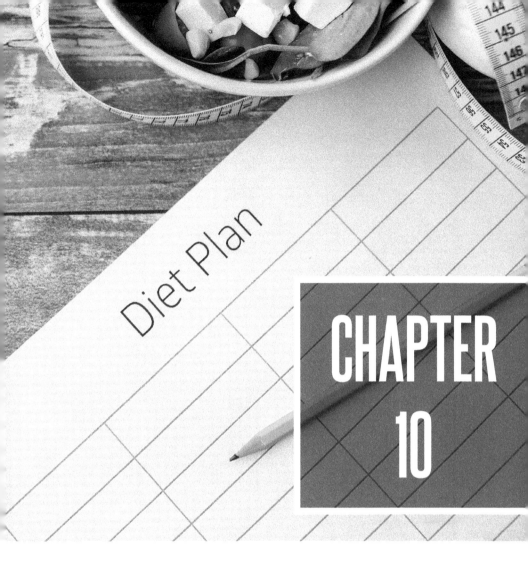

21 DAY MEAL PLAN

Chapter 10 - 21 Day Meal Plan

If you'd rather rely on your own skills to make your Keto-friendly menu, think about how to make the process even more efficient for yourself. While some people enjoy cooking every single day, others don't have the time for it. Meal prepping can help you greatly. If you can devote a single day to your grocery shopping and meal prepping, then you can likely save a lot of time when it comes to how much cooking must be done. Try to plan your menus ahead of time, taking note of recipes that sound interesting and healthy. When you have these ideas in advance, you are likely going to be able to make faster decisions in the grocery store.

Use your meal prep time as a time to unwind. Even if cooking isn't your favorite thing to do, know that you are doing this because you are making an investment towards your health. Prepare and store all of the food that you will need for the week, dividing it into portion-controlled containers. Ideally, you should sort all of the food by meal type. This way, you will be able to simply grab a portion and go or heat it when you need to eat something. Many Keto meal prep recipes can be eaten either hot or cold, which is helpful when you are at the office or anywhere else away from your home. You might find that the whole family will become interested in your newfound meal prep ways.

If you do want to get the entire family involved in meal planning, this serves as a great way to bond and work together to come up with the plan. Eating healthy can be difficult for many reasons, but when given options, it makes the process a lot easier. Show your family the recipes you've come up with and the ones that you have grown to love. Even if they are not on the Keto diet themselves, it is highly likely that they will find your meals just as delicious as you do. Keep a recipe book handy and add new recipes to it as you see them. When you are constantly keeping track of them, you will be more likely to remember them for later.

Remember that you can utilize a mix of both eating out and cooking for yourself when you are on Keto. The key is to take a look at your lifestyle and your current schedule in order to determine what is going to work best for you. Meal prepping can be a gradual process, so if you are only able to prep for a few days at a time, try it out this way. Nothing about eating should have to be an all or nothing process. The important thing is to pay attention to your body. If you notice that you don't feel as energized when you eat at restaurants, then you are likely not getting enough nutrition. The best way to truly give your body what it needs is by preparing the food yourself. When you can listen to your body, you will always know what you need next.

Day	Breakfast	Lunch	Dinner	Snack
1	Bacon Cheeseburger Waffles	Green Beans Salad	Korma Curry	Keto Cheesecakes
2	Keto Breakfast Cheesecake	Apple Salad	Zucchini Bars	Keto Brownies
3	Egg-Crust Pizza	Asian Salad	Mushroom Soup	Raspberry and Coconut
4	Breakfast Roll-Ups	Octopus Salad	Stuffed Portobello Mushrooms	Chocolate Pudding Delight
5	Basic Opie Rolls	Shrimp Salad	Lettuce Salad	Peanut Butter Fudge
6	Almond Coconut Egg Wraps	Lamb Salad	Onion Soup	Cinnamon Streusel Egg Loaf
7	Bacon & Avocado Omelet	Coconut Soup	Asparagus Salad	Snickerdoodle Muffins

8	Bacon & Cheese Frittata	Broccoli Soup	Beef with Cabbage Noodles	Yogurt and Strawberry Bowl
9	Bacon & Egg Breakfast Muffins	Simple Tomato Soup	Roast Beef and Mozzarella Plate	Sweet Cinnamon Muffin
10	Bacon Hash	Green Soup	Beef and Broccoli	Nutty Muffins
11	Bagels With Cheese	Sausage and Peppers Soup	Garlic Herb Beef Roast	Pumpkin and Cream Cheese Cup
12	Baked Apples	Avocado Soup	Sprouts Stir-fry with Kale, Broccoli, and Beef	Berries in Yogurt Cream
13	Baked Eggs In The Avocado	Avocado and Bacon Soup	Beef and Vegetable Skillet	Pumpkin Pie Mug Cake
14	Banana Pancakes	Roasted Bell Peppers Soup	Beef, Pepper and Green Beans Stir-fry	Chocolate and Strawberry Crepe

v	Breakfast Skillet	Spicy Bacon Soup	Cheesy Meatloaf	Blackberry and Coconut Flour Cupcake
16	Brunch BLT Wrap	Taco Stuffed Avocados	Roast Beef and Vegetable Plate	Keto Cheesecakes
17	Korma Curry	Buffalo Shrimp Lettuce Wraps	Breakfast Roll-Ups	Keto Brownies
18	Zucchini Bars	Keto Bacon Sushi	Basic Opie Rolls	Raspberry and Coconut
19	Mushroom Soup	Keto Burger Fat Bombs	Almond Coconut Egg Wraps	Chocolate Pudding Delight
20	Stuffed Portobello Mushrooms	Caprese Zoodles	Bacon & Avocado Omelet	Peanut Butter Fudge
21	Lettuce Salad	Zucchini Sushi	Bacon & Cheese Frittata	Cinnamon Streusel Egg Loaf

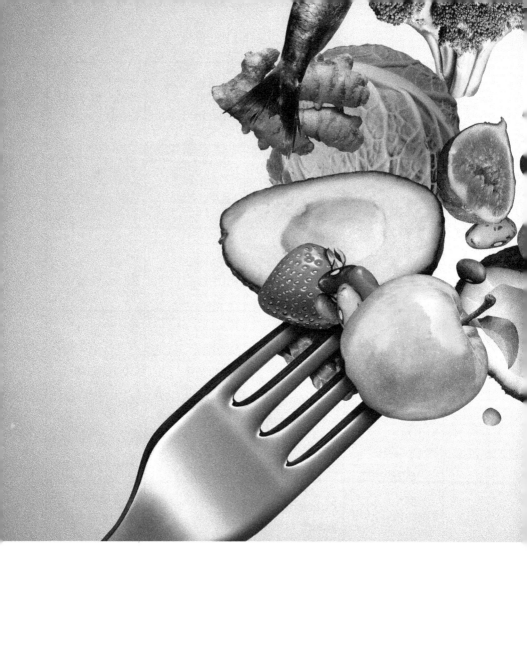

CHAPTER 11

WHY IS IT IMPORTANT TO STICK TO THE KETOGENIC MEAL PLAN?

Chapter 11 - Why Is It Important to Stick to the Ketogenic Meal Plan?

We have tackled this topic several times in this guidebook already. However, the question 'why is it important to stick to the Ketogenic diet' keeps coming up all the time. As we stated earlier, the Ketogenic diet has numerous benefits to you once you have decided to start on it. Let us find an answer to this recurring question.

THE KETOGENIC DIET IS IMPORTANT BECAUSE:

It reduces your blood's insulin and sugar levels; if you have diabetes, the Ketogenic diet is very helpful. Doing away with carbohydrates is proven to reduce your blood sugar levels drastically. This also reduces your insulin levels in the blood. This is, however, efficient if you have visited and consulted with your doctor, and they have suggested the

Ketogenic meal plan for you. This diet could even remedy type 2 diabetes.

It lowers your body's blood pressure: Hypertension is a great risk factor to you because you could contact other diseases such as stroke, kidney failure, or even heart-related diseases. However, sticking to the Ketogenic diet could prove itself beneficial because doing away with carbohydrates lowers your blood pressure and thus reduces your chances of contracting the diseases mentioned above and could assist you in living longer.

It improves your LDL Cholesterol levels: If you have high LDL cholesterol levels, you stand a great risk of contracting heart-related diseases, including possible heart attacks. This depends on the particle size of the LD. If you have large particles, then your chances of suffering from a heart attack are low, while having small particles increases your risk of suffering from a possible heart attack. The Ketogenic diet increases the LDL particles in size in your blood. Thus, if you opt to lower your consumption of carbohydrates, you are improving your chances of avoiding a possible heart attack.

It is a therapy for brain disorders: Glucose is very important for your brain in its day to day functioning. Your brain burns glucose to provide energy for it to function normally. Once you adopt the Ketogenic diet, your body's liver is forced to produce glucose from the protein you ingest. However, your brain can also burn ketones, which are a result of the Ketogenic diet. This way, the diet remedies epilepsy in children who are unresponsive to the drugs related to epilepsy. The diet could be a possible cure for epilepsy. The diet is also known for its ability to remedy Alzheimer's disease as well as Parkinson's disease.

It lowers your body's triglycerides: If you are wondering what triglycerides are, they are fat molecules that move in your blood. It has been proven that high levels of triglycerides could lead to heart-related diseases. These levels are elevated in your body if you consume high amounts of carbohydrates, and thus, the diet comes in handy and assists you to cut on your carbs consumption. Additionally, consuming low fats could also raise the levels of triglycerides in your blood, which makes the Ketogenic diet appropriate to stick to.

This diet is an effective agent in your attempts to lose weight. You are cutting carbohydrates in your diet in the most effective way for you to lose weight. Low carb diets are very effective in weight loss because of their ability to get rid of excess water in your body in the process lowering your body's insulin levels, which in turn speeds up your weight loss. This is, however, effective in short-term weight loss and not so effective for the long-term plan. This is why it is important to seek your physician's opinion before embarking on the diet.

It reduces your appetite: The Ketogenic diet is important in reducing your appetite if you are trying to fight obesity. Hunger is what leads to overeating and becoming obese in the end. Cutting carbohydrates in your meal and ingesting more fats and proteins leads to consuming fewer calories. Doing away with carbohydrates is one way to minimize your appetite as well as your intake of calories.

In conclusion, if you are looking to boost your blood's sugar and insulin levels or if you are looking to lose appetite, lose weight, lower your triglycerides, remedying brain disorders, lowering your blood pressure or becoming healthier in general, you have all the reasons to stick to the diet.

How Long Would It Take for the Ketogenic Diet to Be Effective?

By now, you already know that the Ketogenic diet is among the world's famous low carbohydrates diet. The diet is responsible for the reason why your body no longer burns carbohydrates; instead, it burns fats to produce ketones that are responsible for the day to day functioning of your body. After adopting the diet, the question 'how long until you enter ketosis' begs for attention. Most people get worried that they might not enter ketosis in time, and thus, they tend to give up on a diet as a result.

The fact is that the amount of time it would take you to enter ketosis is not the same amount of time someone else could need to get into ketosis. Additionally, many people find it hard for their bodies to enter ketosis. Let us take a look at how long it could take you to enter ketosis.

For you to benefit from the diet, your body needs to get into ketosis first. Ketosis, as we defined it earlier, is a state that your body adapts to when it starts burning fats into molecules, which we referred to as ketones. Ketones are your body's main source of energy once your body stops burning carbohydrates to produce glucose, usually the main source of energy on the normal diet.

The first step that you would take as a way of reaching ketosis is doing away with carbohydrates. It is important to note that your body stores excess glucose in your liver or your muscles. The glucose is stored in its storage form, glycogen. Switching to burning fats by your body could take time because your body would be required to burn all the glucose in your body before opting to burn fats for energy. The time required for your body to successfully make this change is different from everyone else. This could be because of varying carbohydrates intake in your daily meals as well as varying consumptions of proteins, fats, or how regularly you exercise your body, your age, or even your body's metabolism rates.

For instance, if you consume carbohydrates at high or elevated levels, once you have started on the Ketogenic diet, your body could take longer before it gets into ketosis. This is contrary to your consumption of carbohydrates as an average or lower consumer. It would take you a shorter time compared to the high levels of carbohydrates consumers to get into ketosis. This is because your body would be required to finish all its glucose in the body, including the stored glycogen. The more carbohydrates you consume, the more the stored glycogen and the more the amount of time required to burn it in your body completely.

It would require you between 2 to 5 days, if you are an average consumer of carbohydrates, to get into ketosis. This is approximate if you consume 50 to 60 grams of carbohydrates in a day. The duration of time could be altered depending on several factors, including; the body's metabolism, your age, your level of physical activity as well as your protein, carbohydrates, and fat intake.

You would be able to tell if you are on ketosis if you experienced a number of symptoms, including the Ketogenic flu. You could experience nausea, bad breath, elevated thirst, or fatigue. These are possible ways to tell if you are already on ketosis. However, the most accurate and reliable source of knowledge on your ketosis level is if you test your body of the ketone levels. You could opt to visit your doctor or physician, and they would run a few tests on you to determine the ketone levels in your body. Or you could measure the

Beta-hydroxybutyrate levels using the ketone meter at the comfort of your house.

Some people take longer to get into ketosis because they most probably ingest carbohydrates without knowing. Consuming carbohydrates could hinder the rate at which it would require your body to get into ketosis. It could as well get your body out of ketosis in the process. There is no standard limit to limit your consumption of carbohydrates to ensure that your body gets into ketosis. Different people could get into ketosis by eating different levels of carbohydrates you included. This is why it is important to consult with your doctor. Another possible reason could be that you are not ingesting the required levels of fats in your diet. The Ketogenic advocates for up to 70% of fats to be consumed as well as 20% of protein and possibly 5% or 10% of carbohydrates. Changing or altering this ratio could mean you will take longer to get into ketosis. Other reasons could be your age, physical exercise levels, personal stress, or even lack of adequate sleep. These could affect the rate at which your body could get into ketosis.

You could improve your chance of getting into ketosis if you exercise regularly, minimize your carbohydrates consumption, increase your fat consumption, or even by testing your ketone levels regularly.

Chapter 12 - Cheating On the Ketogenic Diet

We will look at cheating on a diet. The occasional slip up happens in all diets, and you shouldn't feel bad for it if it does. Let it go and get back on track as soon as possible. However, you should always try to avoid excessive binges or cheat days.

So, let's talk about cheating. Can you have cheat meals on the keto diet?

It is normal among dieters to factor in a once a week 'cheat meal' that allows them some slack and gives them something to look forward to food-wise. However, the keto diet isn't just a diet. It's a lifestyle and one that tends to be stricter than the majority of low-carb diets. What this means is that if you have a cheat meal, it can have a higher impact on your progress than for other diets.

To get a grip on just how cheating on a ketogenic diet can affect you, let's take a look at the disadvantages of cheat meals.

Cheating, even just once, can make you leave a state of ketosis. This is even more true if you eat something that is loaded with carbs. Why

229

is it so easy to leave ketosis? Remember, your body will naturally want to use glucose as an energy source, purely because it's easy to produce. The minute you fill your body with carbs, you flood your system with easy-to-use glucose. It will then take you some time to get back into ketosis because you need to wait for the glucose supplies to leave your body. Measure your ketone levels if you are concerned after eating a specific meal.

To make your body start burning fat for fuel involves a complex metabolic process. The side effects you may feel in the initial stages of going on the keto diet are the result of your body using new hormones and adjusting the production of certain enzymes to help burn fat. By eating cheat meals, it prevents your body from completing this process, and consequently, from staying in ketosis. In the long run, this means you won't be burning fat, and you'll have to restart the process all over again.

The keto diet is great for those with diabetes, as it helps control the level of glucose in the blood. Eating a cheat meal loaded with carbs counters this benefit and causes spikes in your blood sugar levels. Not only does this cancel out the positives of the keto diet, but it can also be dangerous.

Cheating will cause cravings. Just as you're getting used to the healthy, wholesome food on the keto diet, the minute you eat something off the menu, it kickstarts your prior attachment to that food and will make you want more. It may leave you having to readjust to eating low-carb again.

Remember how the keto flu can kick in during the beginning stages of the keto diet? By having cheat meals, your body has to readapt to burning fat instead of glucose, which can bring on those symptoms of the keto flu again. These unpleasant effects include headaches, fatigue, and generally feeling run down.

So, what do you do if you want to do the keto diet, but the idea of not having a cheat meal seems way too restrictive? The good news is that although it is better to follow the keto diet as strictly as possible, some alternatives will cut you a bit of slack.

How to Cheat Sensibly On the Keto Diet

First things first, to get the most out of the ketogenic diet, it's best to follow it as strictly as possible. If you do slip up and eat carbs once in a while, don't be harsh on yourself. In the grand scheme of things, one off-moment will make little difference. It's when it becomes regular that it starts to become a concern.

If you want to incorporate a few cheat meals into your ketogenic diet, then here are the best ways to do it. It will slow down the process compared to following the keto diet strictly, but you will still be making progress and reaping the health benefits of the keto diet. There are two main options:

There is a kind of keto diet known as the CKD or the Cyclical Ketogenic Diet. Monday to Friday, for example. Then, on the weekend, you can normally eat with carbs. This doesn't mean you should pile on the carbs, but it allows certain treats like the odd glass of wine and wholemeal bread. The downside is this will probably take you out of ketosis. The good news is, it still gives some health benefits, preserves muscle mass, and helps make the diet far easier to stick to.

The other option is to stick to your keto diet, and instead of making the cheat meal loaded in carbs, make the cheat meal one that is relatively keto-friendly and that you will enjoy. Don't cheat because you are driven to binge for emotional reasons. Try to identify why you want to cheat on the diet and try to find a healthy substitute for what you are craving. For example, if you want pizza, make one with almond flour, which is far better on the keto diet. This will help to avoid binging and craving more non-friendly keto food after.

It can't be said enough, though – the best form of the keto diet is when you follow it properly. This will bring you the highest number of health benefits, and you will feel great for it.

So, what happens if you've been following it correctly and then suddenly, you have one slip up?

GETTING BACK INTO KETOSIS AFTER CHEATING

Firstly, be kind to yourself. Sometimes, cheating is not exactly 'cheating.' Eating an entire doughy pizza is, unfortunately, cheating, but eating something that is not exactly perfect for keto is fine now and again. Keto is a lifestyle, not something to make you feel guilty or miserable. Try doing the best you can, and if you eat the occasional pack of popcorn at the cinema or biscuit with your coffee, let it go and keep the focus on your keto diet for the rest of the day.

Don't rationalize your cheat meal with the idea that now that you have created, you may as well just carry on for the rest of the day. Instead, after a cheat, make that your last one, as this will reduce the time it takes to get back in ketosis. A one-day binge can take a few days to get back into ketosis. A one-off cheat will be much easier and quicker to get back on track, and you may find that you are still in a state of ketosis.

After a cheat, make sure your next foods are high in fat and very low in carbs and low in proteins. This will help balance the effect and make getting back into ketosis a bit easier.

If you have eaten a high-carb snack or meal, try doing some exercise afterward. A walk is fine, but the best thing to do is to do an intensive weight lifting or high-intensity workout session. This will help use up that glucose in your system and force your body to use the glycogen stored up in the muscles. By doing this, you will return to ketosis much quicker or even manage to stay in ketosis.

Plan as much as possible and figure out when and why you cheat. This will help you know what to do in these situations. For example, do you find yourself snacking on junk food when you are out? In that case, try taking keto-snacks with you wherever you go. Maybe you get cravings at certain times of the month, especially for women on hormonal cycles. Figure out what it is you are craving and prepare a similar yet keto-friendly substitute for these kinds of moments.

After a cheat meal, drink lots and lots of water. This will help you feel full and help you only eat again when you are genuinely hungry.

Just because one day you had lots of extra calories, it doesn't mean you should eat fewer calories the next day. The idea is to keep eating nutritious food to ward off cravings and remain healthy.

Don't worry if you get out of ketosis. Try to avoid this happening, of course, but keep your morale high – you will be back in it again soon. Most of all, don't beat yourself up over it. The worst thing you can do is demotivate yourself by making yourself feel guilty. Draw a line under it and move on.

Try to remember why you started the keto diet in the first place. Use that to reconsider your relationship with food. Your body doesn't need loads of carbs to survive, and thinking of food as eating to live the best life you can give your body rather than living to eat can help you get a perspective the next time you fancy something carb-filled or sugary.

Chpater 13 - Sustainable Weight Loss on the Ketogenic Diet

While weight loss is fairly simple while following the Ketogenic Diet, the real kicker is keeping the weight off! The key here is to remember that the Ketogenic Diet is meant to be a change in lifestyle, not just another yo-yo diet for you to quit again.

If you have lost weight in the past just to gain it all back within a year or two, you are not alone! Below, you will find some of the best keto hacks that will help you lose weight and keep it off in the long run.

KEEP IT SIMPLE, STUPID

In the modern world, there are a million and one ways to lose weight. Most of these methods work at first, but as soon as people lose weight, they stop putting in the work! The issue here is that the diet is just not sustainable. The ketogenic diet will change all that, as long as you are doing it correctly.

When you first begin any diet, you are probably all in and getting results from it. The key here is to keep going once you have accomplished your goals! The only way to stick with a diet is to make sure that you are enjoying it. If you are being too restrictive or too stressed out about what you are eating, there is no way you can do this for a long period!

Instead, try to stick to the basic roots of the Keto diet and stop being so hard on yourself. You have a thorough understanding of what you can and cannot eat. Eat low carbs, avoid sugar, and enjoy the fat. When you follow these simple rules, you will drop weight in no time! There is absolutely no reason to make this diet harder than necessary. You will want to strive for progress, not perfection.

If you slip up? Who cares! You will want to be mindful of your mistake and then get right back on your horse! One slip up is not going to ruin all of your progress. So, what if you get kicked out of ketosis for the day? There is always the next day and the day after that. You will want to try to avoid getting stuck on one mistake. We are human; we eat bad things every once in a while. As long as you are not eating junk every day, you will still lose weight! Stop making it complicated.

SET GOALS YOU CAN REACH

While it may seem like the Ketogenic Diet is a miracle worker, you will still want to set realistic goals for yourself. When you set goals that you can't reach, this can be very discouraging. As you begin your new journey, remember that there are going to be many struggles along the way. You may have seen crazy success stories on social media, but you do not know the work that went into those changes. Weight loss is not going to happen overnight, and it certainly did not happen for anyone. For this reason, set realistic goals and be easy on yourself.

As you set goals for yourself, remember that slow and steady wins the race! When you begin the Keto Diet, your body is going through much change, just like you are. Instead of striving to lose the thirty pounds at once, try setting a more realistic goal of one to two pounds a week! This type of goal is both realistic and sustainable.

With that in mind, stop comparing yourself to other people! While following your new diet, you are going to see many success stories. You are not these individuals; you do not have their genes; you do not have their struggles, stop comparing yourself! Instead, I invite you to use your past self as motivation. If you are fat, sick and dying, change your life! Use the Ketogenic Diet to improve yourself, not to be better than other people.

One final note for setting goals is not to allow yourself to obsess over your progress. It is natural to be curious about your weight daily, but what you need to know if that your weight is going to fluctuate, no matter how good you are about your diet! I suggest tracking once every other week. If your results are not moving in the right direction after a month, that is when you can make changes to your diet. You are allowed to track your progress, just don't obsess over the numbers!

CHANGE YOUR FOOD ENVIRONMENT

In the beginning, your motivation and willpower are enough to help you transform your health, but for many individuals, this is not enough to help maintain results. In the long run, many people return to their old habits and gain the weight back. If you want to kick this habit, you must change your lifestyle, not just your diet! Luckily for you, there are some simple strategies you can use to lose weight and keep it off.

One of the major things you will need to do when starting a new diet is to change your environment! You will want to create a safe space that feeds your results instead of your body! When you think about it, many of us eat when we are emotional. When we are emotional, the brain kicks into a gear telling you that you need to satisfy a craving, but then the rational part of you says you need to stick with your diet! No matter how motivated or strong-willed you are, many give in to the cravings at some point. This emotional environment is what influences weight gain in the first place. To avoid this, it is time to change your food environment!

REMOVE THE CARBS

The first step you will need to take is to remove any food item that is high in carbs or unhealthy from your home. You already know what you can eat, get rid of anything that is not on your list! By removing these items, you will be able to get rid of the trigger itself and avoid reaching for it when the cravings hit you hard.

Once that is complete, go ahead and store your healthy foods in more convenient places. When the healthier options are more accessible, you will reach for these to help fuel your body instead of dragging it down. When you eat healthier and have only healthy options, you are increasing the chances you'll stick with your diet!

HAVE A PLAN

Just because you are on a diet does not mean that you cannot enjoy the foods you are eating; you just have to be smarter about your options! Cravings are unavoidable, that is just a fact of life. Instead of crying about it and wishing you could dive into your favorite snack, come up with a keto-friendly plan! There are some incredible keto-desserts out there to satisfy your sweet tooth. When you do cave to a crave, just be sure to keep it in moderation!

MAKE KETO-ADAPTION EASIER

Starting the Keto Diet is going to be a very exciting time, but expect to hit your first speed bump fairly quickly. When you start restricting carbs, you are going to send your body into a total whirlwind. Remember that this process involves losing electrolytes, shedding water weight at a rapid pace, and shifting your hormone levels. As your body throws a tantrum over losing carbohydrates, you will start your keto-flu, which may take away your newfound excitement fairly quickly.

While the keto-flu is no joke, remember staying hydrated is going to be key here to help simmer down the symptoms. However, there are also ways other than carb restriction that you can help your body transition into ketosis in an easier manner. Below, you will find some keto hacks to help you out with your progress on the Ketogenic Diet.

MCTs

If you are a ketogenic beginner, do yourself a favor and invest in quality MCT oils. These medium-chain triglycerides will help increase the ketone levels in your body and reduce the amount of time it takes to get into ketosis. Less time getting into ketosis means less time for the keto flu to bring you down! The best part is that all it takes is 1-2 tablespoons a day! If this is your first time, you will want to start with a lower dose. For beginners, MCT can cause some stomach discomfort. Either way, MCT is a great secret tool to have in your kitchen!

EXERCISE

No matter how old you are, there are all different types of exercises that can help increase the ketone production in your body. If you are looking to increase fat burning, low-intensity exercises will be a great option for you. If you are looking for a more intense workout such as HITT or weightlifting, this can also help deplete your glycogen levels and increase the production of ketones. The key here is to move your body! In the second book of this series, you will be provided with not only delicious recipes to fuel your new diet, but also a series of exercises to kick your body right into ketosis!

Ultimately, your success on your new diet is going to be completely in your hands. While this guidebook is here to give you all the tips and tricks you need to get started, this guidebook isn't going to hand the results to you! The Ketogenic Diet does take some work and effort, but the benefits make it worthwhile. If you are willing to give it time, you will lose the weight and keep it off. How well you do is going to be up to you.

Chapter 14 - Conclusion

Your dedication to improve your health and lose weight is phenomenal since you have been able to reach the end of this guidebook. It is not an easy process to lose weight if you will be able to maintain the guidelines you have learned in this guidebook and stay motivated; your life will change in ways that you cannot imagine. You are on the right track to achieve both mental and physical health. Even though adjusting to eating a healthy diet after being accustomed to eating a lot of convenience foods is a challenge, you will feel the difference in energy levels that you will experience. You will look good and be safe from many of the common nutrition-related diseases and conditions and on top of all of that, your quality of life will improve greatly.

We are all different thus, you should take time to really understand what a weight loss program involves and try out the program gradually. If you nose dive into a weight loss program is not advisable since it may not be for you. No regiment works perfectly for everyone thus, you should select a plan and modify it in a way that suits you. There are many weight loss programs with mind-blowing results, but they may be too hard to follow or just unsafe to practice.

You work out intensity, duration, your resting period are all factors that should be considered. It best works when it is a constant in your daily activity and as it is not a permanent change of your physical and psychological condition.

In order to get the maximum weight loss experience, you should listen to your body. This does not mean that you should eat any time you feel hungry, it means that you should listen to how it responds to your diet and fasting regiment because the body system determines the time for you to eat, time for you to exercise and even how many calories you take in. Thus you will be in full control of your weight loss once you are in control of your diet and fasting program.

You should know that even though the ketogenic diet is about carbohydrate restriction, do not excessively restrict them, you should make sure you eat enough. If you restrict calories too much, you will be moody and it can even stop your fat loss process. You should also vary your food choices so that you make sure that you are getting the nutrients you need to maintain your health.

In fact, getting all the nutrients that you require from a ketogenic diet is possible. Unfortunately for some, this is not possible. If you do not feel okay, you should go and see a doctor to determine if you have any nutritional deficiencies. He/she will able to recommend supplements for you from that information.

For health reasons, weight loss should be a slow process. Losing 2 pounds a day is okay, but anything more than that is a lot. Engage in your day-to-day operations while fasting as this is a time-flying route. Good luck with your keto diet journey!

KETO DIET COOKBOOK

AFTER 50

A Specific Cookbook To
Rapid Weight Loss, Get A
Better Metabolism, Burn
Fat, Control Diabetes,
Get A Ketogenic
Body And Boost
Your Energy With
A Tasty Meal
Plan

Over 80 easy recipes

ALICE HARWING

KETO DIET COOKBOOK AFTER 50

A comprehensive guide to get a better metabolism, burn fat, lose weight prevent diabetes, get a ketogenic body and boost your energy with a tasty meal plan

ALICE HARWING

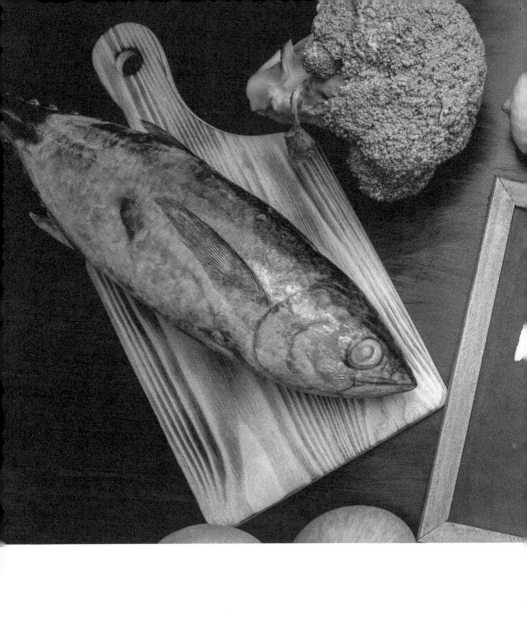

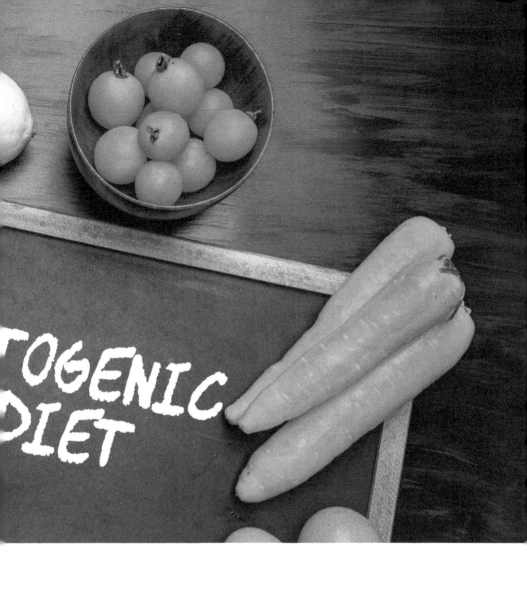

INTRODUCTION

Introduction

When **you start at about** 50, you will notice a lot of changes in your body, it is more than normal. Among the most common symptoms, there is a loss of muscle, insomnia, finer skin. You don't have to worry about this, but you have to pay much more attention than usual to your lifestyle, it is essential, to keep fit, that you start attending a gym, as well as a healthy and correct diet under all macros.

You can apply it even if you have health problems. Of course, a visit to a nutritionist can help you personalize your diet even more effectively. But this is "something more," the information in this guidebook is more than enough, you just need to study it and apply it diligently.

As said, the functions of our body change according to age, in particular, the thing that changes most is our metabolism, it is physiological that it slows down with age. This change is due both to aging, but also to our lifestyle. Current metabolism is a consequence of our lifestyle in recent years.

A healthy lifestyle, with frequent low-abundance meals, with moderate alcohol consumption, will certainly have a faster metabolism than a lifestyle consisting of large meals eaten once a day, alcohol, and insomnia.

The ketogenic diet can definitely help you from this point of view, eliminating carbohydrates and promoting the elimination of fats from our body. Another advantage is its flexibility, in fact, you can play with macros and adapt them to your needs and your lifestyle, in addition to the progress made, of course.

Start gradually, your body has adapted for years to an unhealthy lifestyle, so do not overdo it overnight. Take your time and slowly reach your goals. There is no need to run, this is a marathon, not 100 meters.

At first, you may feel tired, tired, without energy. Don't worry, it's a normal thing, it's your body that is adapting to the new food style. You're taking away its main source of energy, carbohydrates, it's logical that it has to adapt. It must change the main energy source, it must switch to using fats, but this takes time, two or three days are necessary. The drop in sugars could decrease your pressure for a couple of days, avoid exercise and there will be no problems. The resulting benefits will be enormous.

Consult a nutrition specialist. This guidebook is a very valuable tool to get an idea of what a ketogenic diet is, what the benefits are, how to avoid classic mistakes. It is a complete guide, with which, if studied well, you will certainly be able to set your diet according to your daily needs. However, consulting a doctor is never a bad idea, you can discuss your opinions and can give you valuable advice. I recommend consulting your doctor, especially in cases of health problems and in cases where you have never been on a diet.

INTRODUCTION

This book is filled with delicious keto meals that you can cook in your own home. The recipes in this book are easy to do and complete with preparation time, cooking time, ingredients, directions, and nutritional facts. Read on and let's get started.

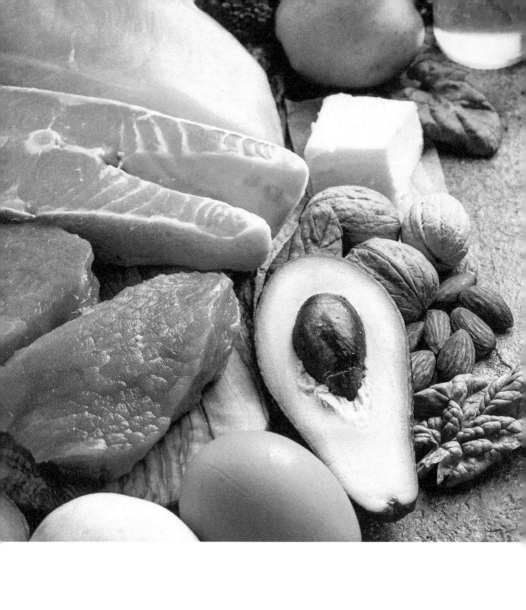

CHAPTER 01

WHAT IS A KETOGENIC DIET

Chapter 01 - What Is A Ketogenic Diet

You are going to receive a glimpse into what the keto weight-reduction plan sincerely is and how it stacks up relative to the other famous diets obtainable on the market. This sort of comparative evaluation would be capable of doing things. One, it will let you gather perspective on the weight loss plan enterprise and the variety of alternatives that might have a purpose worth trying. And, it will offer you a more informed opinion and a more strong resolve for whatever healthy diet weight-reduction plan you do eventually pick to adopt for yourself inside the future.

KETO AS THE BEST DIET PLAN OUT THERE

It's proper that there are undoubtedly many weight loss plan plans obtainable at the market, and it'd be too arrogant to say that the keto weight loss plan is high-quality among them all. However, it would be fair to mention that the keto eating regimen is a high-quality one for you for my part if it takes place to serve your wishes and your goals higher effectively.

The keto food plan is a low-carb diet that is designed to place the human frame into a heightened ketogenic state, which might inevitably result in higher pronounced fat burn and weight loss. It is a reasonably accessible food regimen with a variety of keto-friendly meals being readily available in marketplaces at highly low prices. It isn't an eating regimen that is reserved most effectively for the affluent and elite.

As some distance as effectiveness is concerned, there's just no denying how impactful a keto eating regimen might be for someone who wants to lose a drastic quantity of weight in a wholesome and managed manner. The keto weight-reduction plan also enforces discipline and precision for the agent by incorporating macro counting and meal journaling to ensure accuracy and accountability in the weight-reduction project. There are no external factors that can impact how robust this weight loss plan may be for you. Everything is all within your control.

And lastly, it's a reasonably sustainable weight loss plan, for the reason that it doesn't merely compromise on taste or range. Sure, there are lots of restrictions. But ultimately, there are lots of alternatives and workarounds that can assist stave off cravings. If these kinds of standards and reasons observe to you and your personal life, then it could genuinely be safe to say that the keto food plan is a high-quality one for you.

WHAT SETS KETO APART FROM OTHERS?

But how precisely does keto stack up against other weight loss plan plans obtainable? Well, if your purpose for dieting is weight loss, then it would be prudent to investigate different diets that are similar to the keto eating regimen's goals of inducing weight reduction and fats burn. You should advantage a higher understanding of these diets and why the keto eating regimen would, in all likelihood, nonetheless be the better one for you. The three foods which are most usually compared to the keto weight loss plan in phrases of meal composition and bodily effects are Atkins, paleo, and Whole30.

ATKINS

The Atkins and keto diets are so similar in the feel that they both promote a high intake of fat, mild consumption of protein, and minimum intake of carbohydrates. Typically, while on Atkins, a person's typical diet would be composed of 60% fat, 30% protein, and 10% carbohydrates. This is still a relatively minimal carbohydrate composition even when you take into consideration the keto breakdown of 75% fat, 20% protein, and 5% carbohydrates.

The problem with Atkins isn't found in better carbohydrate consumption. It's, in most cases, located inside the elevated consumption of protein. Any extra protein that the body doesn't dissipate for muscle constructing or repair is converted into glucose. And that glucose goes to be used for energy in preference to the stored fat that you could have, at this moment making the metabolic fee of your frame slower. The keto diet nonetheless offers you the protein blessings of constructing and repairing muscles without compromising the advantages of ketosis at the same time.

PALEO

The paleo food regimen is one that is gaining full-size popularity in the cutting-edge health industry. It stems from the studied nutritional practices of the Paleolithic era, which was depending on the hunter-gatherer system of food rationing and production. It is a food regimen that focuses entirely on complete ingredients that are free from any processing. Food items which include wheat, grains, dairy, legumes, processed sugars, processed oils, corn, processed fats, etc. are prohibited. It specializes in the high intake of meats and non-starchy greens.

Like the keto weight-reduction plan, the paleo diet additionally takes place to be a low-carb diet that emphasizes a better consumption of fat and proteins. However, it doesn't indeed restrict the wide variety of carbohydrates or energy that a person might take on day by day basis. It's a weight loss plan that focuses entirely on the composition of meals without the quantity of it, and that may be problematic for several people who've very particular bodily composition dreams.

WHOLE30

Whole30 is a stricter model of the paleo weight-reduction plan. It is a diet plan that is primarily dependent on a thirty-day application of strict eating under paleo principles. It removes the consumption of processed foods, starchy vegetables and carbohydrates, sweeteners, dairy products, legumes, and higher. Once the thirty-day period is over, you're then recommended to reintroduce certain food groups step by step in your weight-reduction plan and examine what kind of impact or effect these will have on you. This is how you will be capable of discovering what type of food you've got a trendy intolerance to.

However, the Whole30 weight loss program doesn't certainly issue in macro counting and calorie counting either. That manner that humans at the Whole30 weight loss plan are nevertheless at risk of gaining weight and getting fat despite the restrictive nature of the weight loss program.

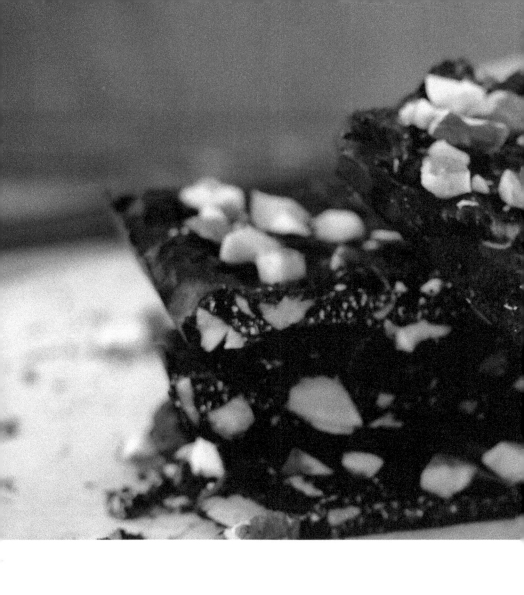

CHAPTER 02

WHAT YOU CAN'T EAT ON A KETO DIET

Chapter 02 - What You Can't Eat On A Keto Diet

will show you the kinds of food you want to avoid at all costs. Because keto is a keto diet, that means you need to avoid high-carbs food. Some of the food you avoid is even healthy, but they just contain too many carbs. Here is a list of common food you should limit or avoid altogether.

BREAD AND GRAINS

Bread is a staple food in many countries. You have loaves, bagels, tortillas, and the list goes on. However, no matter what form bread takes, they still pack many carbs. The same applies to whole-grain as well because they are made from refined flour.

Depending on your daily carb limit, eating a sandwich or bagel can put you way over your daily limit. So if you want to eat bread, it is best to make keto variants at home instead.

Grains such as rice, wheat, and oats pack many carbs as well. So limit or avoid that as well.

FRUITS

Fruits are healthy for you. They have been linked to a lower risk of heart disease and cancer. However, there are a few that you need to avoid in your keto diets. The problem is that some of those foods pack quite a lot of carbs such as banana, raisins, dates, mango, and pear.

As a general rule, avoid sweet and dried fruits. Berries are an exception because they do not contain as much sugar and are rich in fiber. So you can still eat some of them, around 50 grams. Moderation is key.

VEGETABLES

Vegetables are just as healthy for your body. Most of the keto diet does not care how many vegetables you eat so long as they are low in starch. Vegetables that are rich in fiber can help with weight loss. For one, they make you feel full for longer, so they help suppress your appetite. Another benefit is that your body would burn more calories to break and digest them. Moreover, they help control blood sugar and aid with your bowel movements.

But that also means you need to avoid or limit vegetables that are high in starch because they have more carbs than fiber. That includes corn, potato, sweet potato, and beets.

PASTA

Pasta is also a staple food in many countries. It is versatile and convenient. As with any other convenient food, pasta is rich in carbs. So when you are on your keto diet, spaghetti or any other types of pasta are not recommended. You can probably get away with it by eating a small portion, but that is not possible.

Thankfully, that does not mean you need to give up on it altogether. If you are craving pasta, you can try some other alternatives that are low in carbs such as spiralized veggies or shirataki noodles.

CEREAL

Cereal is also a huge offender because sugary breakfast cereals pack many carbs. That also applies to "healthy cereals." Just because they use other words to describe their product does not mean that you should believe them. That also applies to oatmeal, whole-grain cereals, etc.

So when you eat a bowl of cereal when you are doing keto, you are already way over your carb limit, and we haven't even added milk into the equation! Therefore, avoid whole-grain cereal or cereals that we mention here altogether.

BEER

In reality, you can drink most alcoholic beverages in moderation without fear. For instance, dry wine does not have that many carbs, and hard liquor has no carbs at all. So you can drink them without worry. Beer is an exception to this rule because it packs a lot of carbs.

Carbs in beers or other liquid are considered to be liquid carbs, and they are even more dangerous than solid carbs. You see, when you eat food that is rich in carbs, you at least feel full. When you drink liquid carbs, you do not feel full as quickly, so the appetite suppression effect is little.

SWEETENED YOGURT

Yogurt is very healthy because it is tasty and does not have that many carbs. It is a very versatile food to have in your keto diet. The problem comes when you consume yogurt variants that are rich in carbs such as fruit-flavored, low-fat, sweetened, or nonfat yogurt. A single serving of sweetened yogurt contains as many carbs as a single serving of dessert.

If you love yogurt, you can get away with half a cup of plain Greek yogurt with 50 grams of raspberries or blackberries.

JUICE

Fruit juices are perhaps the worst beverage you can put into your system when you are on a keto diet. One may argue that juice provides some nutrients, but the problem is that it contains many carbs that are very easy to digest. As a result, your blood sugar level will spike whenever you drink it. That also applies to vegetable juice because of the fast-digesting carbs present.

Another problem is that the brain does not process liquid carbs the same way as solid carbs. Solid carbs can help suppress appetite, but liquid carbs will only put your appetite into overdrive.

Low-Fat and Fat-Free Salad Dressings

Fruits and vegetables are largely okay, so long as they are low in carbs. But if you have to buy salads, keep in mind that commercial dressings pack more carbs than you think, especially the fat-free and low-fat variants.

So if you want to enjoy your salad, dress your salad using creamy, full-fat dressing instead. To cut down on carbs, you can use vinegar and olive oil, both of which are proven to help with heart health and aid in weight loss.

BEANS AND LEGUMES

These are also very nutritious as they are rich in fiber. Research has shown that eating these have many health benefits, such as reduced inflammation and heart disease risk.

However, they are also rich in carbs. You may be able to enjoy a small amount of them when you are on your keto diet, but make sure you know exactly how much you can eat before you exceed your carb limit.

SUGAR

We mean sugar in any form, including honey. You may already be aware of what foods that contain lots of sugar, such as cookies, candies, and cake, are forbidden on a keto diet or any other form of diet that is designed to lose weight.

What you may not be aware of is that nature's sugar, such as honey, is just as rich in carbs as processed sugar. Natural forms of sugar contain even more carbs.

Not only that sugar, in general, is rich in carbs, they also add little to no nutritional value to your meal. When you are on a keto diet, you need to keep in mind that your diet is going to consist of food that is rich in fiber and nutritious. So sugar is out of the question.

If you want to sweeten your food, you can just use a healthy sweetener instead because they do not add as many carbs to your food.

CHIPS AND CRACKERS

These two are some of the most popular snacks. What some people did not realize is that one packet of chips contain several servings and should not be all eaten in one go. The carbs can add up very quickly if you do not watch what you eat.

Crackers also pack many carbs, although the amount varies based on how they are made. But even whole-wheat crackers contain many carbs.

Due to how processed snacks are produced, it is difficult to stop yourself from eating everything within a short period. Therefore, it is advised that you avoid them altogether.

MILK

Cereal contains many carbs, and a breakfast cereal will put you way over your carbs limit without you adding milk. Milk also contains many carbs on its own. Therefore, avoid it if you can even though milk is a good source of many nutrients such as calcium, potassium, and other B vitamins.

Of course, that does not mean that you have to ditch milk altogether. You can get away with a tablespoon or two of milk for your coffee. But cream or half-and-half is better if you drink coffee frequently. These two contain very few carbs. But if you love to drink milk in large amounts or need it to make your favorite drinks, consider using coconut milk or unsweetened almond instead.

GLUTEN-FREE BAKED GOODS

Wheat, barley, and rye all contain gluten. Some people who have celiac disease still want to enjoy these delicacies but unable to because their gut will become inflamed in response to gluten. As such, gluten-free variants have been created to cater to their needs.

Gluten-free diets are very popular nowadays, but what many people don't seem to realize is that they pack quite a lot of carbs. That includes gluten-free bread, muffins, and other baked products. In reality, they contain even more carbs than their glutenous variant. Moreover, the flour used to make these gluten-free products are made from grains and starches. So when you consume a gluten-free bread, your blood sugar level spikes.

So, just stick to whole foods. Alternatively, you can use almond or coconut flour to make your low-carb bread.

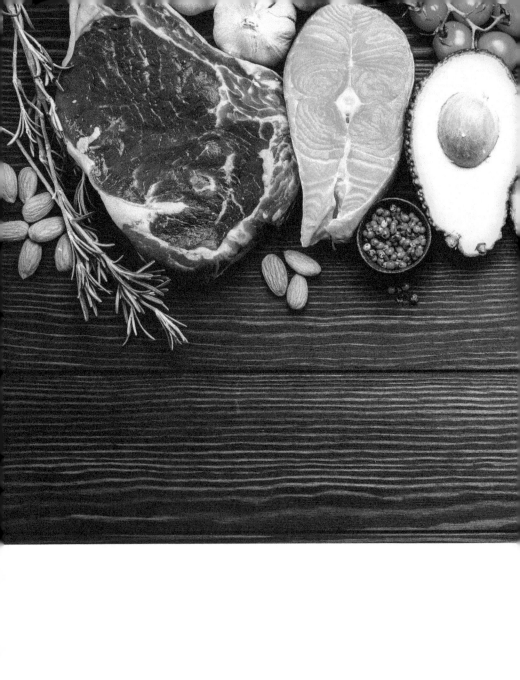

ALLOWED
PRODUCT LIST

Chapter 03 - Allowed Product List

FATS

Your daily consumption of fats will be around 70% of your food intake. This needs to be high-quality fat that stays in your system to be used as energy. These are typically found in fats that are the result of raw foods and animals.

Some of the best fats for keto are:

- Hard Cheeses
- Nuts like almonds, walnuts, pecans, and macadamia
- Seeds from sunflowers, pumpkins, chia, flaxseed and hemp hearts
- Natural oils like olive oil and coconut oil
- The cacao of at least 85% cacao. This must be unsweetened and unprocessed chocolate
- Poultry, especially dark meat
- Fatty fish
- Whole eggs, especially the yolks
- Whole milk produces like whole milk mozzarella and ricotta
- Cheese

When we look at high-fat foods, cheese tops the list. It is high in fat and has no carbohydrates. Unfortunately, cheese contains many calories, along with unhealthy saturated fats. When you are consuming cheese, be mindful of the amount you eat. Some cheese is a healthy snack and a good alternative to chips and sugary snack items. Small amounts of cheese in your diet, a few ounces daily, will help you control your hunger because it is filling. It has also been found that calcium in cheese may have a positive effect on blood pressure and cholesterol. Consumption of cheese has also been found to increase muscle mass.

NUTS

As you choose which nuts you're going to eat on keto, be sure to take note of the net carbs. Some nuts have more fat than others, and some have more calories and carbohydrates than others. Choose nuts that will fit well in your macros. Because of the high calories and carbs eat nuts in moderation. They may also have a significant amount of protein when eating a large quantity. Be sure you are adhering to your protein macros as well as your carbohydrate macros.

SEEDS

The good thing about seeds about keto is that the carbohydrates are mostly offset by fiber. That makes the net carbohydrates friendly for keto. Seeds tend to be high in fat and contain some protein. However, they often contain harmful omega-6 fatty acids. You can benefit from the normal concentration of nutrients in seeds, but eating them sprouted. To sprout seeds, simply germinate the seeds between two wet paper towels and leave them to sit for 2 to 8 days. Make sure your paper towel remains moist. Eventually, the stem will sprout from the seed. It's still high in nutrients but easier to digest.

OILS

Oils can be your best cooking aid in the keto diet. They must be able to burn at high temperatures to be most effective for cooking. It is important to use unsaturated fats to provide the most heart-healthy oils. The polyunsaturated oils will be a good addition to the fats consumed on a keto like nut oils and avocado oils. These will assist you in achieving a healthy, effective keto diet. Avocado oil, sesame oil, coconut oil, and olive oil have essential qualities to aid in digestion and nutrient absorption. Also, coconut oil speeds up metabolism.

MEAT/FISH/EGGS/DAIRY

Unprocessed meats do not contain carbohydrates, and many are high in fat. Grass-fed meats are better than grain-fed but watch the portion size. Be careful not to exceed the protein requirements in your daily macros. Fish is good, especially fish high in fat like salmon. Avoid the breading, which has carbohydrates. Again, wild-caught fish is better. It is fed naturally off of foods fish are accustomed to eating. This reduces the chance that growth hormones and antibiotics may be included in the feed from farm fat raised fish. Along the same lines, try to stick to cage-free pasture-raised eggs in the hopes of avoiding chemical additives that might reduce the quality of the food you are consuming. The same is true for milk. Milk and dairy products should be organic to avoid growth hormones and antibiotics that may be found in conventional Foods today. Meat fish eggs and dairy are high in fat; I can be a good source of the fat you need to consume on the keto diet.

PROTEINS

Protein will make up 20% of your daily food intake. It is important not to exceed your protein macros. Be sure you're making good decisions regarding your protein if a person that you are including your diet. It will be consuming a lot of fat, which may contain much protein. So you have to be sure to combine your fat macros with your protein macros when you're setting up your meal plan for the day.

Some of the proteins that you will be eating that are most efficient are:

- Salmon
- Mackerel
- Tuna
- Sardines
- Eggs
- Greek yogurt

- Shrimp
- Chicken thighs
- Peanuts
- Pistachios
- Almonds
- Soybeans (edamame)

NUT BUTTER

The goal of the keto diet is not to eat low-fat proteins. Luckily, there are many high-fat proteins available for consumption. Many times, you will be able to satisfy your fat macros and protein macros with the same food items. Watch your calories, and be sure to incorporate your snack foods into your protein count. Be mindful that green leafy vegetables also contain protein.

It is important to consume enough protein so that carbohydrates in your body do not use muscle to convert to energy. Conversely, too much protein can cause muscle tissue to break down and turn into sugar because of the lack of carbohydrates available on a low-carb diet. Eat the right amount of protein, and don't forget about adding in the protein found snacks and vegetables, especially cream hidden ones when considering your protein macros.

FISH

Some of the best foods for protein on keto are fatty proteins found in salmon, mackerel, and sardines. These proteins are high in fat and omega-3 fatty acids. Fresh fish is higher in omega-3 fatty acid than canned fish, but if you are going to eat fish protein, make sure it is high in fat. This is an efficient way to consume protein and fat that will be converted to energy.

EGGS

Some studies indicate that people who include dairy in their diet have less hunger, and the consumption of dairy may inhibit the production of cortisol, and therefore, the resulting abdominal fat. Full-fat dairy is high in calories, so be sure not to over-consume. It is common for conventional milk and dairy products to contain growth hormones. Dairy from grass-fed animals and organic dairy products are recommended. Aside from the hormones, conventional dairy products do not have as high levels of omega-3 fatty acids, which have anti-inflammatory qualities and promote joint health. Dairy contains much protein. If you're eating meat protein, you should be especially cognizant of the amount of dairy that you're eating so you do not exceed your protein macros. Egg whites are lower in calories and contain the protein of the egg. The egg yolks contain the fat of eggs. If you're going to eat meat and eggs and you have consumed enough fat for the daily macro, you may be able to eat the white instead of the yolks without adding additional fat. The yolk also carries the bulk of calories from eggs, and egg whites have very few calories.

NUTS/NUT BUTTERS/SOYBEANS

Nuts and soybeans (edamame) make excellent snack foods on keto. Eating good quality protein and protein-filled snacks, especially after exercising, may assist your body in building muscle. Snacks should be kept small. They should simply be a means to curb your hunger pains. That is why a quick snack of nuts is ideal. They contain some proteins, some fats, and some carbohydrates. Count the nuts you select to be sure you don't eat too many carbs. Carefully measure the serving size of your snack. Since nuts are small, it is easy to think that eating a few extra nuts here and there won't matter. Whether this is true depends on the nut. That's a good way to add moderate levels of protein to your diet and to adjust your protein macros for the day.

CARBOHYDRATES

So far, it has been stressed to eat more fat, the correct amount of protein, and now, it is time for carbohydrates. Eat fewer carbohydrates. Consume 10% of your daily food in the form of carbohydrates.

This is the crux of the ketogenic diet. Normally, carbohydrates are limited to 5% of the daily calories eaten. In doing the gentle keto, the carbohydrates are increased to 10%. Whether 5% or 10%, be sure to minimize the number of carbohydrates in your diet. Also, try to make the carbohydrates of good quality that will burn off quickly so that your body moves quickly to burning fat.

There are many no-carb options available when eating fats and protein. What is needed to add to your diet are vegetables. Produce has nutrients and vitamins that your body needs, so they should be included in your diet. Be sure to incorporate foods that have valuable nutrients such as vegetables and berries into your diet. These are low in carbohydrates. Some of the vegetables and fruits should be used more sparingly than others. Look at green leafy vegetables and vegetables that grow above the ground as low carbohydrate options to provide healthy options that will not add fat. Vegetables that grow underground like carrots and potatoes tend to have more sugar content and are higher in carbohydrates.

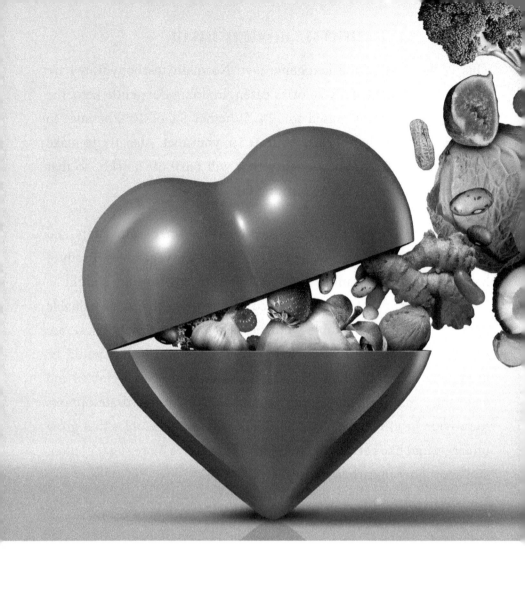

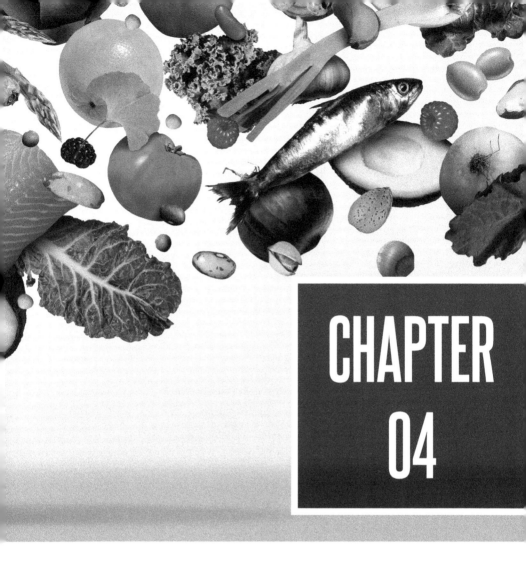

CHAPTER 04

THE FOODS THAT CAN HELP TO SLOW DOWN AGING

Chapter 04 - The Foods That Can Help To Slow Down Aging

Your food intake for the day should be as clean as possible because this can help you to get a youthful look. Consider looking into whole foods diets such as Paleo, Juicing, or Plant-Strong, since these are simple to follow and will give you the basics of how to cut out processed and toxin-filled junk. Most of these diets are not expensive despite what you may think and you might actually find yourself saving money as well as losing weight. Whole foods are good because they're often much more filling than junk and because they're rich in all the anti-aging nutrients you could possibly need. In fact, if you're using a food tracker, simply eating cleaner may mean you won't even need a multivitamin or some anti-aging supplements (like high-dose Vitamin C). If at all possible, get your nutrients from your food, they're better quality and much easier for the body to absorb than the pharmaceutical versions. Remember that calorie restriction is important when it comes to eating well for anti-aging.

At the end of your day, head home to another nutritious meal, but don't forget to spend time with people that you care about. Being present in your life will make it much more meaningful, what's the point in living 100 years if you don't enjoy it? By being social and present, you'll also get the anti-aging benefits of doing so as well as create better memories for yourself. Consider getting together to do something active as you'll need to be up and moving at least 30 minutes a day. If you haven't yet done your yoga consider looking into partner-yoga or classes together. Partner yoga is an ideal way to bring you closer together too. If possible, try to do this in places of nature. Being around nature has been proven to have a positive impact on the brain.

If you're going to head to the gym, try and find one that has a sauna. The reason for this is that sweating is one of the most efficient ways for your body to get rid of toxins. Cigarette smoke and sun damage can all age your skin through toxins, but these are quickly sweated out in a sauna. Studies have shown that by using a sauna regularly, you can help reduce the appearance of wrinkles temporarily. As the steam penetrates the skin, the pores open up, releasing anything in the cells to the steam. You'll only need to spend 10-20 minutes in there to feel the beneficial effects.

Don't forget your supplement regime throughout the day. Many anti-aging supplements need to be taken at specific times or with meals, so plan your supplements accordingly and consider getting a pill organizer if you can't remember them.

When you finally head to bed, you'll want to make sure that you're moisturizing your skin again. If you didn't make your 8 glasses of water, consider having one before bed to top up what you've missed. A hot cup of tea is also an ideal way to relax before bed. Lavender oil has many anti-aging properties and is also great for relaxation. You can take lavender as a relaxing tea before bed or put a few drops of the oil onto your pillow before going to bed.

The key to being successful in this plan is that you need to be able to fit as many of these things into your daily routine as possible. It's fairly established that if you can do something for 7 days, then it will become a hàbit, so simply trying to do it for that long before saying you can't is important. But, above all, if you didn't make your 8 glasses, haven't done your yoga, or ate that hamburger – Don't stress about it! A little slip now and then happens, so let it go and remember that tomorrow is another day.

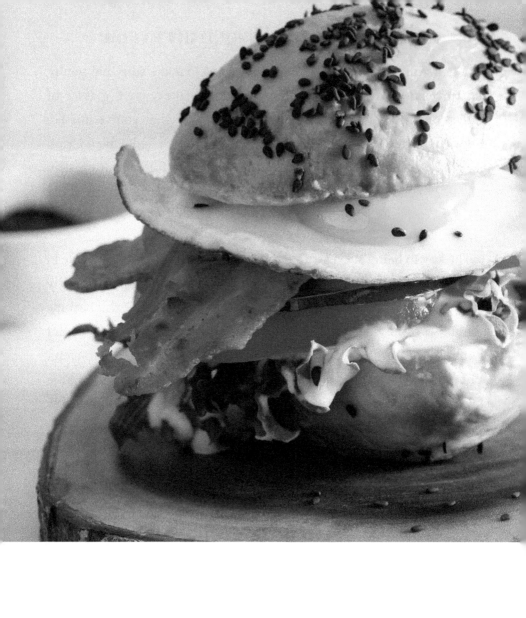

CHAPTER 05

BREAKFAST

Bacon Cheeseburger Waffles

PREPARATION
10 MINS

COOKING
20 MINS

4 SERVINGS

INGREDIENTS

- Toppings

- Pepper and Salt to taste

- 1.5 ounces of cheddar cheese

- 4 tablespoons of sugar-free barbecue sauce

- 4 slices of bacon

- 4 ounces of ground beef, 70% lean meat and 30% fat

- Waffle dough

- Pepper and salt to taste

- 3 tablespoons of parmesan cheese, grated

- 4 tablespoons of almond flour

- ¼ teaspoon of onion powder

- ¼ teaspoon of garlic powder

- 1 cup (125 g) of cauliflower crumbles

- 2 large eggs

- 1.5 ounces of cheddar cheese

NUTRIRION

- Fats: 12g
- Calories: 152g

- Proteins: 6g
- Carbohydrates: 3g

DIRECTIONS

1. Preheat oven to around 350 degrees F.

2. Pulse almonds in a food processor then add in butter and sweetener.

3. Pulse until all the ingredients mix well and coarse dough forms.

4. Coat twelve silicone muffin pans using foil or paper liners.

5. Divide the batter evenly between the muffin pans then press into the bottom part until it forms a crust and bakes for about 8 minutes.

6. In the meantime, mix in a food processor the cream cheese and cottage cheese then pulse until the mixture is smooth.

7. Put in the extracts and sweetener then combine until well mixed.

8. Add in eggs and pulse again until it becomes smooth; you might need to scrape down the mixture from the sides of the processor. Share equally the batter between the muffin pans, then bake for around 30-40 minutes until the middle is not wobbly when you shake the muffin pan lightly.

9. Put aside until cooled completely, then put in the refrigerator for about 2 hours and then top with frozen and thawed berries.

KETO BREAKFAST CHEESECAKE

PREPARATION
20 MINS

COOKING
45 MINS

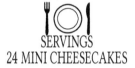
SERVINGS
24 MINI CHEESECAKES

INGREDIENTS

- Toppings

- 1/4 cup of mixed berries for each cheesecake, frozen and thawed

- Filling ingredients

- 1/2 teaspoon of vanilla extract

- 1/2 teaspoon of almond extract

- 3/4 cup of sweetener

- 6 eggs

- 8 ounces of cream cheese

- 16 ounces of cottage cheese

- Crust ingredients

- 4 tablespoons of salted butter

- 2 tablespoons of sweetener

- 2 cups of almonds, whole

NUTRIRION

- Fats: 12g

- Calories: 152g

- Proteins: 6g

- Carbohydrates: 3g

DIRECTIONS

1. Preheat oven to around 350 degrees F.

2. Pulse almonds in a food processor then add in butter and sweetener.

3. Pulse until all the ingredients mix well and coarse dough forms.

4. Coat twelve silicone muffin pans using foil or paper liners.

5. Divide the batter evenly between the muffin pans then press into the bottom part until it forms a crust and bakes for about 8 minutes.

6. In the meantime, mix in a food processor the cream cheese and cottage cheese then pulse until the mixture is smooth.

7. Put in the extracts and sweetener then combine until well mixed.

8. Add in eggs and pulse again until it becomes smooth; you might need to scrape down the mixture from the sides of the processor. Share equally the batter between the muffin pans, then bake for around 30-40 minutes until the middle is not wobbly when you shake the muffin pan lightly.

9. Put aside until cooled completely, then put in the refrigerator for about 2 hours and then top with frozen and thawed berries.

Egg-Crust Pizza

PREPARATION
5 MINS

COOKING
15 MINS

1-2 SERVINGS

INGREDIENTS

- ¼ teaspoon of dried oregano to taste

- ½ teaspoon of spike seasoning to taste

- 1 ounce of mozzarella, chopped into small cubes

- 6 – 8 sliced thinly black olives

- 6 slices of turkey pepperoni, sliced into half

- 4-5 thinly sliced small grape tomatoes

- 2 eggs, beaten well

- 1-2 teaspoons of olive oil

-

NUTRIRION

- Calories: 363g

- Fats: 24.1g

- Carbohydrates: 20.8g

- Proteins: 19.25g

DIRECTIONS

1. Preheat the broiler in an oven than in a small bowl, beat well the eggs. Cut the pepperoni and tomatoes in slices then cut the mozzarella cheese into cubes.

2. Put some olive oil in a skillet over medium heat, then heat the pan for around one minute until it begins to get hot. Add in eggs and season with oregano and spike seasoning, then cook for around 2 minutes until the eggs begin to set at the bottom.

3. Drizzle half of the mozzarella, olives, pepperoni, and tomatoes on the eggs followed by another layer of the remaining half of the above ingredients. Ensure that there is a lot of cheese on the topmost layers. Cover the skillet using a lid and cook until the cheese begins to melt and the eggs are set, for around 3-4 minutes.

4. Place the pan under the preheated broiler and cook until the top has browned and the cheese has melted nicely for around 2-3 minutes. Serve immediately.

BREAKFAST ROLL-UPS

PREPARATION
5 MINS

COOKING
15 MINS

SERVINGS
5 ROLL-UPS

INGREDIENTS

- Non-stick cooking spray

- 5 patties of cooked breakfast sausage

- 5 slices of cooked bacon

- 1.5 cups of cheddar cheese, shredded

- Pepper and salt

- 10 large eggs

-

NUTRIRION

- Calories: 412.2g

- Fats: 31.66g

- Carbohydrates: 2.26g

- Proteins: 28.21g

DIRECTIONS

1. Preheat a skillet on medium to high heat, then using a whisk, combine two of the eggs in a mixing bowl.

2. After the pan has become hot, lower the heat to medium-low heat then put in the eggs. If you want to, you can utilize some cooking spray.

3. Season eggs with some pepper and salt.

4. Cover the eggs and leave them to cook for a couple of minutes or until the eggs are almost cooked.

5. Drizzle around 1/3 cup of cheese on top of the eggs, then place a strip of bacon and divide the sausage into two and place on top.

6. Roll the egg carefully on top of the fillings. The roll-up will almost look like a taquito. If you have a hard time folding over the egg, use a spatula to keep the egg intact until the egg has molded into a roll-up.

7. Put aside the roll-up then repeat the above steps until you have four more roll-ups; you should have 5 roll-ups in total.

BASIC OPIE ROLLS

PREPARATION
20 MINS

COOKING
35 MINS

SERVINGS
12 ROLLS

INGREDIENTS

- 1/8 teaspoon of salt

- 1/8 teaspoon of cream of tartar

- 3 ounces of cream cheese

- 3 large eggs

NUTRIRION

- Calories: 45

- Fats: 4g

- Carbohydrates: 0g

- Proteins: 2g

DIRECTIONS

1. Preheat the oven to about 300 degrees F, then separate the egg whites from egg yolks and place both eggs in different bowls. Using an electric mixer, beat well the egg whites until the mixture is very bubbly, then add in the cream of tartar and mix again until it forms a stiff peak.

2. In the bowl with the egg yolks, put in 3 ounces of cubed cheese and salt. Mix well until the mixture has doubled in size and is pale yellow. Put in the egg white mixture into the egg yolk mixture then fold the mixture gently together.

3. Spray some oil on the cookie sheet coated with some parchment paper, then add dollops of the batter and bake for around 30 minutes.

4. You will know they are ready when the upper part of the rolls is firm and golden. Leave them to cool for a few minutes on a wire rack. Enjoy with some coffee

ALMOND COCONUT EGG WRAPS

PREPARATION
5 MINS

COOKING
5 MINS

4 SERVINGS

INGREDIENTS

- 5 Organic eggs

- 1 tbsp Coconut flour

- 25 tsp Sea salt

- 2 tbsp almond meal

NUTRIRION

- Carbohydrates: 3 grams

- Protein: 8 grams

- Fats: 8 grams

- Calories: 111

DIRECTIONS

1. Combine the fixings in a blender and work them until creamy. Heat a skillet using the med-high temperature setting.

2. Pour two tablespoons of batter into the skillet and cook - covered about three minutes. Turn it over to cook for another 3 minutes. Serve the wraps piping hot

Bacon & Avocado Omelet

PREPARATION
5 MINS

COOKING
5 MINS

1 SERVINGS

INGREDIENTS

- 1 slice Crispy bacon

- 2 Large organic eggs

- 5 cup freshly grated parmesan

cheese

- 2 tbsp Ghee or coconut oil or butter

- half of 1 small Avocado

NUTRIRION

- Carbohydrates: 3.3 grams

- Protein: 30 grams

- Fats: 63 grams

- Calories: 719

DIRECTIONS

1. Prepare the bacon to your liking and set aside. Combine the eggs, parmesan cheese, and your choice of finely chopped herbs. Warm a skillet and add the butter/ghee to melt using the medium-high heat setting. When the pan is hot, whisk and add the eggs.

2. Prepare the omelet working it towards the middle of the pan for about 30 seconds. When firm, flip, and cook it for another 30 seconds. Arrange the omelet on a plate and garnish with the crunched bacon bits. Serve with sliced avocado.

Bacon & Cheese Frittata

PREPARATION
5 MINS

COOKING
5 MINS

6 SERVINGS

INGREDIENTS

- 1 cup Heavy cream
- 6 Eggs
- 5 Crispy slices of bacon
- 2 Chopped green onions
- 4 oz Cheddar cheese
- Also Needed: 1 pie plate

NUTRIRION

- Carbohydrates: 2 grams
- Protein: 13 grams
- Fats: 29 grams
- Calories: 320

DIRECTIONS

1. Warm the oven temperature to reach 350° Fahrenheit.

2. Whisk the eggs and seasonings. Empty into the pie pan and top off with the remainder of the fixings. Bake 30-35 minutes. Wait for a few minutes before serving for best results

Bacon & Egg Breakfast Muffins

PREPARATION
15 MINS

COOKING
30 MINS

SERVINGS
12

INGREDIENTS

- 8 large Eggs
- 8 slices Bacon
- .66 cup Green onion

NUTRIRION

- Carbohydrates: 0.4 grams
- Protein: 5.6 grams
- Fats: 4.9 grams
- Calories: 69

DIRECTIONS

1. Warm the oven at 350° Fahrenheit. Spritz the muffin tin wells using a cooking oil spray. Chop the onions and set aside.

2. Prepare a large skillet using the medium temperature setting. Fry the bacon until it's crispy and place on a layer of paper towels to drain the grease. Chop it into small pieces after it has cooled.

3. Whisk the eggs, bacon, and green onions, mixing well until all of the fixings are incorporated. Dump the egg mixture into the muffin tin (halfway full). Bake it for about 20 to 25 minutes. Cool slightly and serve.

BACON HASH

PREPARATION
5 MINS

COOKING
10 MINS

SERVINGS
2

INGREDIENTS

- Ingredients:
- 1 Small green pepper
- 2 Jalapenos
- 1 Small onion
- 4 Eggs
- 6 Bacon slices

NUTRIRION

- Carbohydrates: 9 grams
- Protein: 23 grams
- Fats: 24 grams
- Calories: 366

DIRECTIONS

1. Chop the bacon into chunks using a food processor. Set aside for now. Slice the onions and peppers into thin strips. Dice the jalapenos as small as possible.

2. Heat a skillet and fry the veggies. Once browned, combine the fixings and cook until crispy. Place on a serving dish with the eggs

BAGELS WITH CHEESE

PREPARATION
10 MINS

COOKING
15 MINS

SERVINGS
6

INGREDIENTS

- 2.5 cups Mozzarella cheese
- 1.5 cups Almond flour
- 1 tsp. Baking powder
- 2 Eggs
- 3 oz Cream cheese

NUTRIRION

- Carbohydrates: 8 grams
- Fats: 31 grams
- Protein: 19 grams
- Calories: 374

DIRECTIONS

1. Shred the mozzarella and combine with the flour, baking powder, and cream cheese in a mixing container. Pop into the microwave for about one minute. Mix well.

2. Let the mixture cool and add the eggs. Break apart into six sections and shape into round bagels. Note: You can also sprinkle with a seasoning of your choice or pinch of salt if desired.

3. Bake them for approximately 12 to 15 minutes. Serve or cool and store

BAKED APPLES

PREPARATION
10 MINS

COOKING
1 HOUR

SERVINGS
4

INGREDIENTS

- 4 tsp Keto-friendly sweetener.
- .25 cup chopped pecans
- 75 tsp Cinnamon
- 4 large Granny Smith apples

NUTRIRION

- Carbohydrates: 16 grams
- Fats: 19.9 grams
- Protein: 6.8 grams
- Calories: 175

DIRECTIONS

1. Set the oven temperature at 375° Fahrenheit. Mix the sweetener with the cinnamon and pecans. Core the apple and add the prepared stuffing.

2. Add enough water into the baking dish to cover the bottom of the apple. Bake them for about 45 minutes to 1 hour

Baked Eggs In The Avocado

PREPARATION
10 MINS

COOKING
20 MINS

SERVINGS
1

INGREDIENTS

- Half of 1 Avocado

- 1 Egg

- 1 tbsp Olive oil

- Half cup shredded cheddar cheese

NUTRIRION

- Carbohydrates: 3 grams

- Protein: 21 grams

- Fats: 52 grams

- Calories: 452

DIRECTIONS

1. Heat the oven to reach 425° Fahrenheit.

2. Discard the avocado pit and remove just enough of the 'insides' to add the egg. Drizzle with oil and break the egg into the shell.

3. Sprinkle with cheese and bake them for 15 to 16 minutes until the egg is the way you prefer. Serve.

BANANA PANCAKES

PREPARATION
10 MINS

COOKING
15 MINS

SERVINGS
3

INGREDIENTS

- 2 Bananas

- 4 Eggs

- 1 tsp Cinnamon

- 1 tsp Baking powder (Optional

NUTRIRION

- Carbohydrates: 6.8 grams

- Total: 7 grams

- Calories: 157

DIRECTIONS

1. Combine each of the fixings. Melt a portion of butter in a skillet using the medium temperature setting.

2. Prepare the pancakes 1-2 minutes per side. Cook them with the lid on for the first part of the cooking cycle for a fluffier pancake.

3. Serve plain or with your favorite garnishes such as a dollop of coconut cream or fresh berries

BREAKFAST SKILLET

PREPARATION
10 MINS

COOKING
15 MINS

SERVINGS
2

INGREDIENTS

- 1 lb. Organic ground turkey/ grass-fed beef
- 6 Organic eggs
- 1 cup Keto-friendly salsa of choice

NUTRIRION

- Carbohydrates: 3 grams
- Protein: 21 grams
- Fats: 52 grams
- Calories: 452

DIRECTIONS

1. Warm the skillet using oil (medium heat). Add the turkey and simmer until the pink is gone. Fold in the salsa and simmer for two to three minutes.

2. Crack the eggs and add to the top of the turkey base. Place a lid on the pot and cook for seven minutes until the whites of the eggs are opaque.

3. Note: The cooking time will vary depending on how you like the eggs prepared

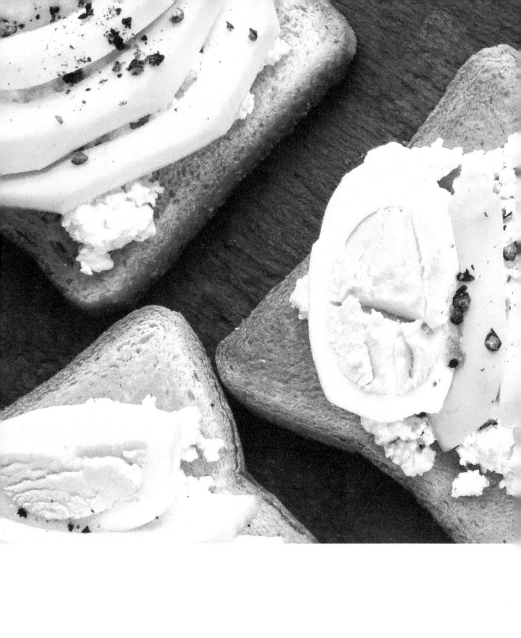

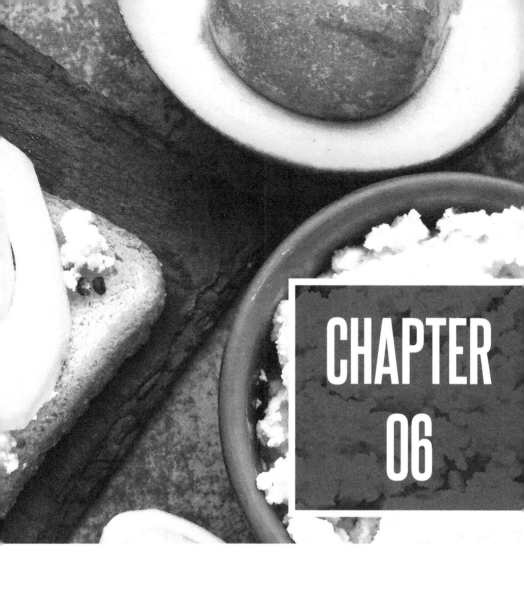

APPETIZERS AND SIDE DISHES

SIMPLE KIMCHI

PREPARATION
10 MINS

COOKING
70 MINS

SERVINGS
4

INGREDIENTS

- 3 tablespoons salt

- 1 pound napa cabbage, chopped

- 1 carrot, julienned

- ½ cup daikon radish

- 3 green onion stalks, chopped

- 1 tablespoon fish sauce

- 3 tablespoons chili flakes

- 3 garlic cloves, peeled and minced

- 1 tablespoon sesame oil

- ½-inch fresh ginger, peeled and grated

NUTRIRION

- Calories: 160

- Fat: 3g

- Fiber: 2g

- Carbohydrates: 5g

- Protein: 1g

DIRECTIONS

1. In a bowl, mix the cabbage with the salt, massage well for 10 minutes, cover, and set aside for 1 hour.

2. In a bowl, mix the chili flakes with fish sauce, garlic, sesame oil, and ginger, and stir well.

3. Drain the cabbage well, rinse under cold water, and transfer to a bowl.

4. Add the carrots, green onions, radish, and chili paste and stir.

5. Leave in a dark and cold place for at least 2 days before serving.

OVEN-FRIED GREEN BEANS

PREPARATION
10 MINS

COOKING
10 MINS

SERVINGS
4

INGREDIENTS

- Ingredients:
- ⅔ Cup Parmesan cheese, grated
- 1 egg
- 12 ounces green beans

- Salt and ground black pepper, to taste
- ½ teaspoon garlic powder
- ¼ teaspoon paprika

DIRECTIONS

1. In a bowl, mix the Parmesan cheese with salt, pepper, garlic powder, and paprika.

2. In another bowl, whisk the egg with salt and pepper. Dredge the green beans in egg, and then in the Parmesan mixture. Place the green beans on a lined baking sheet, place in an oven at 400°F for 10 minutes.

3. Serve hot.

NUTRIRION

- Calories: 114
- Fat: 5g
- Fiber: 7g

- Carbohydrates: 3g
- Protein: 9g

CAULIFLOWER MASH

PREPARATION
10 MINS

COOKING
10 MINS

SERVINGS
2

INGREDIENTS

- ¼ cup sour cream

- 1 small cauliflower head, separated into florets

- Salt and ground black pepper, to taste

- 2 tablespoons feta cheese, crumbled

- 2 tablespoons black olives, pitted and sliced

DIRECTIONS

1. Put water in a pot, add some salt, bring to a boil over medium heat, add the florets, cook for 10 minutes, take off the heat, and drain.

2. Return the cauliflower to the pot, add salt, black pepper, and sour cream, and blend using an immersion blender.

3. Add the black olives and feta cheese, stir and serve.

NUTRIRION

- Calories: 100

- Fat: 4g

- Fiber: 2g

- Carbohydrates: 3g

- Protein: 2g

PORTOBELLO MUSHROOMS

PREPARATION
10 MINS

COOKING
10 MINS

SERVINGS
4

INGREDIENTS

- T12 ounces Portobello mushrooms, sliced

- Salt and ground black pepper, to taste

- ½ teaspoon dried basil

- 2 tablespoons olive oil

- ½ teaspoon tarragon, dried

- ½ teaspoon dried rosemary

- ½ teaspoon dried thyme

- 2 tablespoons balsamic vinegar

DIRECTIONS

1. In a bowl, mix the oil with vinegar, salt, pepper, rosemary, tarragon, basil, and thyme, and whisk.

2. Add the mushroom slices, toss to coat well, place them on a pre-heated grill over medium-high heat, cook for 5 minutes on both sides, and serve.

NUTRIRION

- Calories: 280

- Fat: 4g

- Fiber: 4g

- Carbohydrates: 2g

- Protein: 4g

BROILED BRUSSELS SPROUTS

PREPARATION
10 MINS

COOKING
10 MINS

SERVINGS
4

INGREDIENTS

- 1 pound Brussels sprouts, trimmed and halved

- Salt and ground black pepper, to taste

- 1 teaspoon sesame seeds

- 1 tablespoon green onions, chopped

- 1½ tablespoons sukrin gold syrup

- 1 tablespoon coconut aminos

- 2 tablespoons sesame oil

- 1 tablespoon sriracha

DIRECTIONS

1. In a bowl, mix the sesame oil with coconut aminos, sriracha, syrup, salt, and black pepper, and whisk.

2. Heat a pan over medium-high heat, add the Brussels sprouts, and cook them for 5 minutes on each side.

3. Add the sesame oil mixture, toss to coat, sprinkle sesame seeds, and green onions, stir again, and serve

NUTRIRION

- Calories: 110

- Fat: 4g

- Fiber: 4g

- Carbohydrates: 6

- Protein: 4g

PESTO

PREPARATION
10 MINS

COOKING
0 MINS

SERVINGS
4

- Ingredients

- ½ cup olive oil

- 2 cups basil

- ⅓ cup pine nuts

- ⅓ cup Parmesan cheese, grated

- 2 garlic cloves, peeled and chopped

- Salt and ground black pepper, to taste

DIRECTIONS

1. Put the basil in a food processor, add the pine nuts, and garlic, and blend well. Add the Parmesan cheese, salt, pepper, and the oil gradually and blend again until you obtain a paste. Serve with chicken or vegetables.

NUTRIRION

- Calories: 100

- Fat: 7g

- Fiber: 3g

- Carbohydrates: 1g

- Protein: 5g

Brussels Sprouts and Bacon

PREPARATION
10 MINS

COOKING
30 MINS

SERVINGS
4

INGREDIENTS

- 18 bacon strips, chopped
- 1 pound Brussels sprouts, trimmed and halved
- Salt and ground black pepper, to taste
- A pinch of cumin
- A pinch of red pepper, crushed
- 2 tablespoons extra virgin olive oil

DIRECTIONS

1. In a bowl, mix the Brussels sprouts with salt, pepper, cumin, red pepper, and oil, and toss to coat.

2. Spread the Brussels sprouts on a lined baking sheet, place in an oven at 375°F, and bake for 30 minutes.

3. Heat a pan over medium heat, add the bacon pieces, and cook them until they become crispy.

4. Divide the baked Brussels sprouts on plates, top with bacon, and serve.

NUTRIRION

- Calories: 256
- Fat: 20g
- Fiber: 6g
- Carbohydrates: 5g
- Protein: 15g

CREAMY SPINACH

PREPARATION
10 MINS

COOKING
15 MINS

SERVINGS
2

INGREDIENTS

- 2 garlic cloves, peeled and minced

- 8 ounces of spinach leaves

- A drizzle of olive oil

- Salt and ground black pepper, to taste

- 4 tablespoons sour cream

- 1 tablespoon butter

- 2 tablespoons Parmesan cheese, grated

DIRECTIONS

1. Heat a pan with the oil over medium heat, add the spinach, stir and cook until it softens.

2. Add the salt, pepper, butter, Parmesan cheese, and butter, stir, and cook for 4 minutes.

3. Add the sour cream, stir, and cook for 5 minutes.

4. Divide between plates and serve

NUTRIRION

- Calories: 233

- Fat: 10g

- Fiber: 4g

- Carbohydrates: 4g

- Protein: 2g

AVOCADO FRIES

PREPARATION
10 MINS

COOKING
5 MINS

SERVINGS
3

INGREDIENTS

- 3 avocados, pitted, peeled, halved, and sliced

- 1½ cups sunflower oil

- 1½ cups almond meal

- A pinch of cayenne pepper

- Salt and ground black pepper, to taste

DIRECTIONS

1. In a bowl, mix the almond meal with salt, pepper, and cayenne, and stir. In a second bowl, whisk eggs with a pinch of salt and pepper.

2. Dredge the avocado pieces in egg and then in almond meal mixture. Heat a pan with the oil over medium-high heat, add the avocado fries, and cook them until they are golden.

3. Transfer to paper towels, drain grease, and divide between plates and serve.

NUTRIRION

- Calories: 200

- Fat: 43g

- Fiber: 4g

- Carbs: 7g

- Protein: 17g

ROASTED CAULIFLOWER

PREPARATION
10 MINS

COOKING
25 MINS

SERVINGS
6

INGREDIENTS

- 1 cauliflower head, separated into florets

- Salt and ground black pepper, to taste

- ⅓ cup Parmesan cheese, grated

- 1 tablespoon fresh parsley, chopped

- 3 tablespoons olive oil

- 2 tablespoons extra virgin olive oil

DIRECTIONS

1. In a bowl, mix the oil with garlic, salt, pepper, and cauliflower florets.

2. Toss to coat well, spread this on a lined baking sheet, place in an oven at 450°F, and bake for 25 minutes, stirring halfway. Add the Parmesan cheese, and parsley, stir and cook for 5 minutes.

3. Divide between plates and serve.

NUTRIRION

- Calories: 118

- Fat: 2g

- Fiber: 3g

- Carbohydrates: 2g

- Protein: 6g

Mushrooms and Spinach

PREPARATION
10 MINS

COOKING
10 MINS

SERVINGS
4

INGREDIENTS

- 10 ounces spinach leaves, chopped

- Salt and ground black pepper, to taste

- 14 ounces mushrooms, chopped

- 2 garlic cloves, peeled and minced

- ½ cup fresh parsley, chopped

- 1 onion, peeled and chopped

- 4 tablespoons olive oil

- 2 tablespoons balsamic vinegar

DIRECTIONS

1. Heat a pan with the oil over medium-high heat, add the garlic and onion, stir, and cook for 4 minutes.

2. Add the mushrooms, stir, and cook for 3 minutes.

3. Add the spinach, stir, and cook for 3 minutes.

4. Add the vinegar, salt, and pepper, stir, and cook for 1 minute.

5. Add the parsley, stir, divide between plates, and serve.

NUTRIRION

- Calories: 200
- Fat: 4g
- Fiber: 6g

- Carbohydrates: 2g
- Protein: 12g

COLLARD GREENS WITH TURKEY

PREPARATION
10 MINS

COOKING
135 MINS

SERVINGS
10

INGREDIENTS

- 5 bunches collard greens, chopped
- Salt and ground black pepper, to taste
- 1 tablespoon red pepper flakes
- 5 cups chicken stock
- 1 turkey leg
- 2 tablespoons garlic, minced
- ¼ cup olive oil

DIRECTIONS

1. Heat a pot with the oil over medium heat, add the garlic, stir, and cook for 1 minute.

2. Add the stock, salt, pepper, and turkey leg stir, cover, and simmer for 30 minutes.

3. Add the collard greens, cover pot again, and cook for 45 minutes.

4. Reduce heat to medium, add more salt and pepper, stir, and cook for 1 hour.

5. Drain the greens, chop up the turkey, mix everything with the red pepper flakes, stir, divide between plates, and serve.

NUTRIRION

- Calories: 143
- Fat: 3g
- Fiber: 4g
- Carbohydrates: 3g
- Protein: 6g

EGGPLANT AND TOMATOES

PREPARATION
10 MINS

COOKING
10 MINS

SERVINGS
4

INGREDIENTS

- 1 tomato, sliced

- 1 eggplant, sliced into thin rounds

- Salt and ground black pepper, to taste

- ¼ cup Parmesan cheese, grated

- A drizzle of olive oil

DIRECTIONS

1. Place eggplant slices on a lined baking dish, drizzle some oil and sprinkle half of the Parmesan.

2. Top eggplant slices with tomato ones, season with some salt and pepper, and sprinkle the rest of the cheese over them.

3. Place in an oven at 400ºF, and bake for 15 minutes.

4. Divide between plates and serve hot as a side dish.

NUTRIRION

- Calories: 55
- Fat: 1.1g
- Fiber: 2g
- Carbohydrates: 0.5g
- Protein: 7g

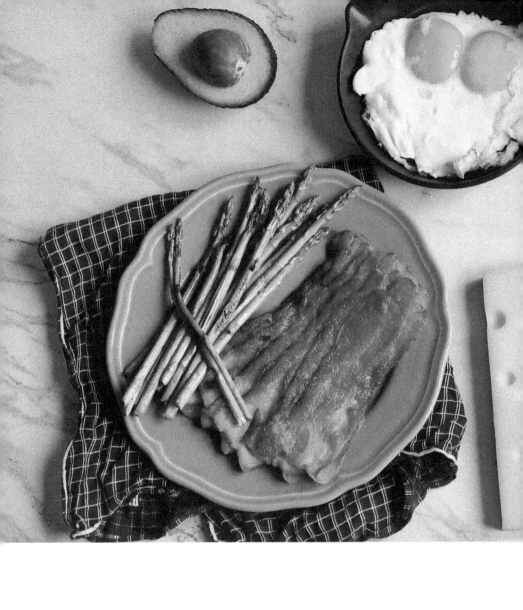

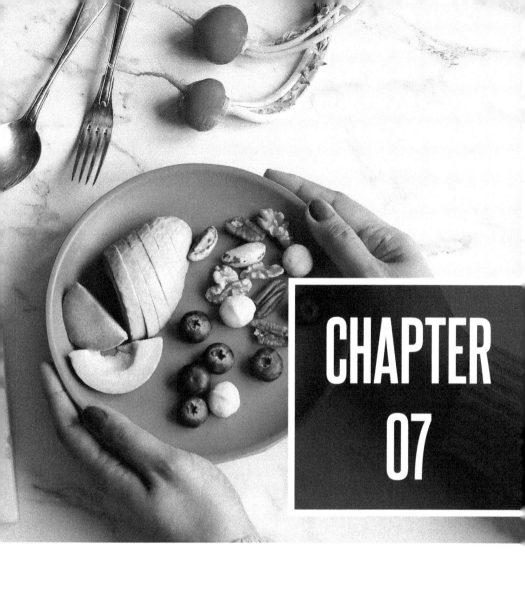

CHAPTER 07

LUNCH

TACO STUFFED AVOCADOS

PREPARATION
12 MINS

COOKING
18 MINS

SERVINGS
6

INGREDIENTS

- 4 Ripe Avocados
- Juice of 1 Lime
- 1 Tbsp. Extra-Virgin Olive Oil
- 1 Medium Onion, Chopped
- 1 Lb. Ground Beef
- 1 Packet Taco Seasoning
- Kosher Salt

- Freshly Ground Black Pepper
- 2/3 Cup Shredded Mexican Cheese
- 1/2 Cup Shredded Lettuce
- 1/2 Cup Quartered Grape Tomatoes
- Sour cream, for topping

NUTRIRION

- Calories: 352
- Carbohydrates: 3.6g

- Fat: 27.4g
- Protein: 22.4g

DIRECTIONS

1. Pit and halve the avocados.

2. With a scoop, scoop out a bit of avocado flesh to create a hole.

3. Dice the removed avocado fresh and set aside for later.

4. Pour lime juice over the avocados to prevent browning.

5. Heat oil in a preheated skillet over medium heat and add chopped onion.

6. Cook the onion until translucent for 3-5 minutes.

7. Stir in ground beef and taco seasoning, breaking up the meat with a wooden spoon.

8. Season the beef with salt and pepper, cook until the meat is browned and no longer pink, about 6 minutes.

9. Turn off the heat and drain the fat, top each avocado half with the cooked beef mixture.

10. Then top with chopped avocado, cheese, lettuce, tomato, and sour cream.

Buffalo Shrimp Lettuce Wraps

PREPARATION
17 MINS

COOKING
23 MINS

SERVINGS
4

INGREDIENTS

- 1/4 Tbsp. Butter

- 2 Garlic Cloves, Minced

- 1/4 C. Hot Sauce, Such as Frank's

- 1 Tbsp. Extra-Virgin Olive Oil

- 1 Lb. Shrimp, Peeled and Deveined, Tails Removed

- Kosher Salt

- Freshly Ground Black Pepper

- 1 Head Romaine lettuce, Leaves Separated, For Serving

- 1/4 Red Onion, Finely Chopped

- 1 Rib Celery, Sliced Thin

- 1/2 C. Blue Cheese, Crumble

NUTRIRION

- Calories: 190

- Carbohydrates: 6g

- Fat: 9.3g

- Protein: 18.1g

DIRECTIONS

1. Pit and halve the avocados.

2. With a scoop, scoop out a bit of avocado flesh to create a hole.

3. Dice the removed avocado fresh and set aside for later.

4. Pour lime juice over the avocados to prevent browning.

5. Heat oil in a preheated skillet over medium heat and add chopped onion.

6. Cook the onion until translucent for 3-5 minutes.

7. Stir in ground beef and taco seasoning, breaking up the meat with a wooden spoon.

8. Season the beef with salt and pepper, cook until the meat is browned and no longer pink, about 6 minutes.

9. Turn off the heat and drain the fat, top each avocado half with the cooked beef mixture.

10. Then top with chopped avocado, cheese, lettuce, tomato, and sour cream

KETO BACON SUSHI

PREPARATION
13 MINS

COOKING
20 MINS

SERVINGS
12

INGREDIENTS

- 6 slices bacon, halved

- 2 Persian cucumbers, thinly sliced

- 2 medium carrots, thinly sliced

- 1 avocado, sliced

- 4 oz. cream cheese softened

- Sesame seeds, for garnish

NUTRIRION

- Calories: 155

- Carbohydrates: 6.7g

- Fat: 12.7g

- Protein: 4.4 g

DIRECTIONS

1. Heat oven to 400 °F (204 °C), line a baking tray with aluminum foil and fit it with a cooling rack.

2. Lay bacon halves in an even layer on the lined baking sheet and place in the oven.

3. Bake until lightly crunchy but still pliable, about 11 to 13 minutes.

4. In the meantime, cut cucumbers, carrots, and avocado into pieces roughly the width of the bacon.

5. Once the bacon is cool enough to touch, spread an even layer of cream cheese on each slice.

6. Divide vegetables evenly between the bacon and place on one end.

7. Roll up vegetables tightly.

8. Garnish with sesame seeds and serve.

9. Enjoy.

KETO BURGER FAT BOMBS

PREPARATION
12 MINS

COOKING
15 MINS

SERVINGS
20

INGREDIENTS

- Cooking spray

- 1 lb. ground beef

- 1/2 tsp. garlic powder

- Kosher salt

- Freshly ground black pepper

- 2 tbsp. cold butter, cut into 20 pieces

- 2 oz. cheddar, cut into 20 pieces

- Lettuce leaves, for serving

- Thinly sliced tomatoes, for serving

- Mustard, for serving

NUTRIRION

- Calories: 77.5

- Carbohydrates: 1.7g

- Fat: 4.8g

- Protein: 6.3g

DIRECTIONS

1. Heat oven to 375 °F (190 °C), grease a mini muffin tin with cooking spray.

2. In a medium bowl, season beef with garlic powder, salt, and pepper.

3. Press one teaspoon beef consistently into the bottom of each muffin tin cup, totally covering the bottom.

4. Place a slice of butter on top then press one teaspoon beef over butter to cover.

5. Place a slice of cheddar on top of meat in each cup then press remaining beef over cheese to cover.

6. Bake the fat bombs until meat is golden and cook through for about 15 minutes.

7. Let cool slightly.

8. Carefully, use a metal offset spatula to release each burger from the tin. Serve with lettuce leaves, tomatoes, and mustard.

9. Enjoy

KETO TACO CUPS

PREPARATION
12 MINS

COOKING
20 MINS

SERVINGS
12

INGREDIENTS

- 2 C. Shredded Cheddar
- 1 Tbsp. Extra-Virgin Olive Oil
- 1 Small Onion, Chopped
- 3 Cloves Garlic, Minced
- 1 Lb. Ground Beef
- 1 Tsp. Chili Powder
- 1/2 Tsp. Ground Cumin
- 1/2 Tsp. Paprika

- Kosher salt
- Freshly ground black pepper
- Sour cream, for serving
- Diced avocado, for serving
- Freshly chopped cilantro, for serving
- Chopped tomatoes, for serving

NUTRIRION

- Calories: 189.8
- Carbohydrates: 1.1g
- Fat: 14.2g
- Protein: 14.2g

DIRECTIONS

1. Preheat oven to 375 °F (190 °C).

2. Line a large baking tray with parchment paper or a baking mat.

3. Put about 2 tablespoons cheddar with a space of 2-inches.

4. Bake the cheese until bubbly and edges turn to golden, about 5-7 minutes.

5. Let the crisps cool on the baking sheet for a minute.

6. Grease bottom of a muffin tin with cooking spray set aside.

7. Put the backed melted cheese slices on the bottom of a muffin tin.

8. Top with another muffin tin and let it cool for 8-10 minutes.

9. Heat oil in a skillet over medium heat, add chopped onion and cook until soft.

10. Add garlic and cook until fragrant, add ground beef, breaking up meat with a spatula.

11. Cook until beef is browned and no longer pink, about 4-6 minutes, then drain the fat.

12. Add meat again to the skillet and season with chili powder, cumin, paprika, salt, and pepper.

13. Place cheese cups on a serving platter.

14. Fill the cheese cups with cooked ground beef and top with sour cream, avocado, cilantro, and tomatoes.

15. Enjoy

CAPRESE ZOODLES

PREPARATION
25 MINS

COOKING
0 MINS

SERVINGS
4

INGREDIENTS

- 4 Large Zucchini
- 2 Tbsp. Extra-Virgin Olive Oil
- Kosher Salt
- Freshly Ground Black Pepper
- 2 C. Cherry Tomatoes Halved

- 1 C. Mozzarella Balls, Quartered If Large
- 1/4 C. Fresh Basil Leaves
- 2 Tbsp. Balsamic Vinegar

NUTRIRION

- Calories: 311
- Carbohydrates: 7.4g
- Fat: 22.2g
- Protein: 16.7g

DIRECTIONS

1. Using a spiralizer, make zoodles out of zucchini.

2. Put zoodles to a big bowl, toss with olive oil and season with pepper and salt.

3. Let marinate 15 minutes.

4. Combine in tomatoes, mozzarella, and basil to zoodles in a bowl and toss until combined.

5. Drizzle with balsamic and serve.

6. Enjoy

Zucchini Sushi

PREPARATION
20 MINS

COOKING
0 MINS

SERVINGS
2

INGREDIENTS

- 2 medium zucchini
- 4 oz. cream cheese softened
- 1 tsp. Sriracha hot sauce
- 1 tsp. lime juice
- 1 c. lump crab meat
- 1/2 carrot, cut into thin matchsticks
- 1/2 avocado, diced
- 1/2 cucumber, cut into thin matchsticks
- 1 tsp. toasted sesame seeds

NUTRIRION

- Calories: 378.8
- Carbohydrates: 10.5g
- Fat: 25.5g
- Protein: 27.7g

DIRECTIONS

1. With a vegetable peeler, slice each zucchini into even thin strips.

2. Place zucchini on a lined plate to dry up the moisture.

3. In a bowl, whisk together cream cheese, Sriracha, and lime juice.

4. Place two zucchini slices down straight on a cutting board.

5. Top with cream cheese in a thin layer on the lift side top with crab, cucumber, and avocado.

6. Roll the zucchini tightly from the lift side.

7. Repeat the process with the remaining zucchini pieces.

8. Garnish with sesame seeds before serving.

ASIAN CHICKEN LETTUCE WRAPS

PREPARATION
13 MINS

COOKING
15 MINS

SERVINGS
4

INGREDIENTS

- 3 tbsp. hoisin sauce

- 2 tbsp. low-sodium soy sauce

- 2 tbsp. rice wine vinegar

- 1 tbsp. Sriracha (optional)

- 1 tsp. sesame oil

- 1 tbsp. extra-virgin olive oil

- 1 medium onion, diced

- 2 cloves garlic, minced

- 1 tbsp. freshly grated ginger

- 1 lb. ground chicken

- 1/2 c. water chestnuts, drained and sliced

- 2 green onions, thinly sliced

- Kosher salt

- Freshly ground black pepper

- Large leafy lettuce (leaves separated), for serving

-

NUTRIRION

- Calories: 280.85

- Carbohydrates: 8.7g

- Fat: 17.6g

- Protein: 21.4g

DIRECTIONS

1. Make the sauce: In a thin bowl.

2. Whisk together hoisin sauce, rice wine vinegar, soy sauce, Sriracha, and sesame oil.

3. In a big skillet over medium-high heat, preheat olive oil.

4. Put onions and cook until soft, about 5 minutes.

5. Then stir in garlic and ginger and cook until fragrant, about 1 minute more.

6. Put ground chicken and cook until opaque and typically cooked through, breaking up meat with a wooden spoon.

7. Pour in the sauce and cook 1 to 2 minutes more, until sauce reduces slightly and chicken cooked through thoroughly.

8. Turn off heat and stir in chestnuts and green onions.

9. Season with pepper and salt.

10. Spoon rice, if using, and a large scoop (about 1/4 cup) of chicken mixture into the center of each lettuce leaf. Serve immediately

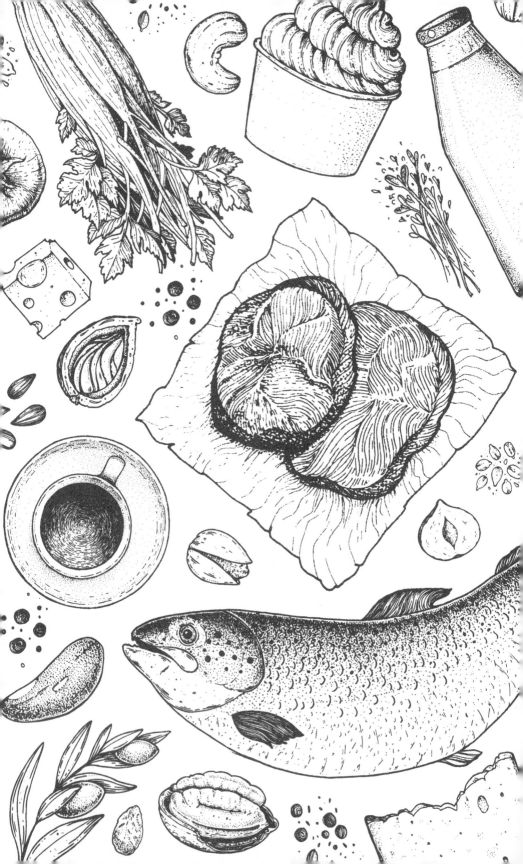

Prosciutto and Mozzarella Bomb

PREPARATION
11 MINS

COOKING
15 MINS

SERVINGS
4

INGREDIENTS

- 4 oz (113g) sliced prosciutto
- 8 oz (226g) fresh mozzarella ball
- Olive oil, for frying
-

DIRECTIONS

1. Coating half of the prosciutto slices vertically.

2. Lay the remaining slices horizontally across the first set of slices.

3. Place your mozzarella ball, upside down, onto the crisscrossed prosciutto slices.

4. Firmly, but very carefully, wrap the mozzarella ball with the prosciutto slices.

5. If making ahead, wrap the balls in cling film and refrigerate.

6. To serve, heat the olive oil in a skillet and crisp the prosciutto on all sides

NUTRIRION

- Calories: 129
- Carbohydrates: 0.3g
- Fat: 11.6g
- Protein: 6.2g

KETOFIED CHICK-FIL-A-STYLE CHICKEN

PREPARATION
14 MINS

COOKING
21 MINS

SERVINGS
8

INGREDIENTS

- 24-oz (680g) pickle jar
- 8 medium uncooked chicken breast tenders
- 4 tbsp almond flour
- ¼ cup grated Parmesan
- Salt and pepper, to taste
- 1 tsp paprika
- 2 large eggs
- 2 tbsp avocado oil

NUTRIRION

- Calories: 407
- Carbohydrates: 12.5g
- Fat: 23.6g
- Protein: 28g

DIRECTIONS

1. In a plastic resealable bag, add the chicken and the pickle juice, marinate in the fridge

2. For 20-30 minutes.

3. On a plate combine the almond flour, grated Parmesan, salt, pepper, and paprika.

4. Whip the eggs together in a separate bowl.

5. Preheat a skillet over medium-high heat and heat the avocado oil.

6. First, dip the chicken pieces in the beaten egg then place it in the breading mixture to coat.

7. Place the chicken into the skillet and cook until golden browned.

CHEESEBURGER TOMATOES

PREPARATION
7 MINS

COOKING
25 MINS

SERVINGS
4

INGREDIENTS

- 1 tbsp. extra-virgin olive oil
- 1 medium onion, chopped
- 2 cloves garlic, minced
- 1 lb. ground beef
- 1 tbsp. ketchup
- 1 tbsp. yellow mustard
- 4 slicing tomatoes

- Kosher salt
- Freshly ground black pepper
- 2/3 c. shredded cheddar
- 1/4 c. shredded iceberg lettuce
- 4 pickle coins
- Sesame seeds, for garnish

NUTRIRION

- Calories: 458
- Carbohydrates: 5g

- Fat: 32.8g
- Protein: 33.4g

DIRECTIONS

1. In a skillet over medium heat, heat oil.

2. Put onion and cook until tender, about 5 minutes, then stir in garlic.

3. Place ground beef, cook and break up the meat with a spatula, cook until the beef browned about 6 minutes, drain fat.

4. Season with salt and pepper, then add the ketch-up and mustard.

5. Flip tomatoes so they are stem-side down.

6. Cut the tomatoes into six wedges, being careful not to cut entirely through the tomatoes.

7. Carefully spread open the wedges.

8. Divide cooked ground beef evenly among the to-matoes.

9. Then top each with cheese and lettuce.

10. Garnish with pickle coins and sesame seeds.

11. Serve it and enjoy it!

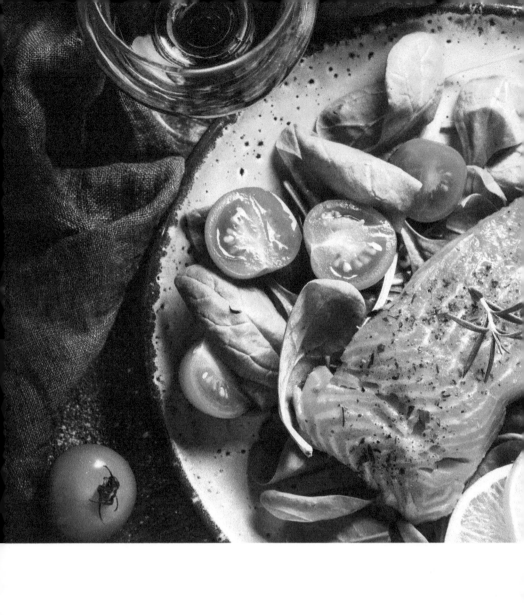

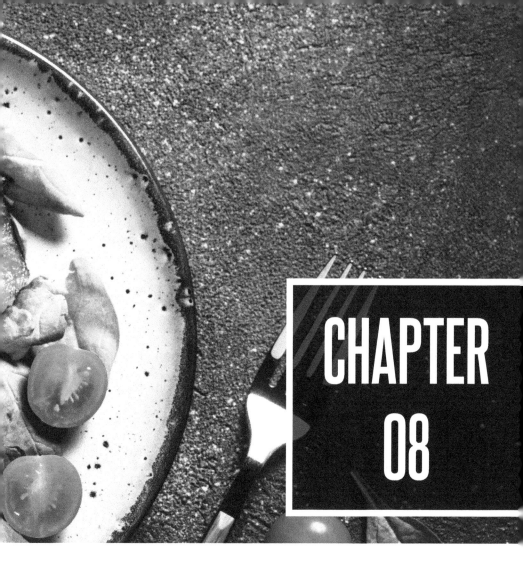

CHAPTER
08

DINNER

KORMA CURRY

PREPARATION
10 MINS

COOKING
25 MINS

SERVINGS
6

INGREDIENTS

- 3-pound chicken breast, skinless, boneless

- 1 teaspoon garam masala

- 1 teaspoon curry powder

- 1 tablespoon apple cider vinegar

- ½ coconut cream

- 1 cup organic almond milk

- 1 teaspoon ground coriander

- ¾ teaspoon ground cardamom

- ½ teaspoon ginger powder

- ¼ teaspoon cayenne pepper

- ¾ teaspoon ground cinnamon

- 1 tomato, diced

- 1 teaspoon avocado oil

- ½ cup of water

NUTRIRION

- Calories: 440

- Fat: 32g

- Fiber: 4g

- Carbohydrates: 28g

- Protein: 8g

DIRECTIONS

1. Chop the chicken breast and put it in the saucepan.

2. Add avocado oil and start to cook it over the medium heat.

3. Sprinkle the chicken with garam masala, curry powder, apple cider vinegar, ground coriander, cardamom, ginger powder, cayenne pepper, ground cinnamon, and diced tomato. Mix up the ingredients carefully. Cook them for 10 minutes.

4. Add water, coconut cream, and almond milk. Saute the meat for 10 minutes more

ZUCCHINI BARS

PREPARATION
10 MINS

COOKING
15 MINS

SERVINGS
8

INGREDIENTS

- 3 zucchini, grated
- ½ white onion, diced
- 2 teaspoons butter
- 3 eggs, whisked
- 4 tablespoons coconut flour
- 1 teaspoon salt
- ½ teaspoon ground black pepper
- 5 oz goat cheese, crumbled
- 4 oz Swiss cheese, shredded
- ½ cup spinach, chopped
- 1 teaspoon baking powder
- ½ teaspoon lemon juice

NUTRIRION

- Calories: 187.2
- Total Fat: 7.3 g
- Saturated Fat: 0.6 g
- Cholesterol: 17.6 mg
- Sodium : 29.5 mg
- Potassium: 74.2 mg
- Total Carbohydrate: 29.5 g
- Protein: 1.7 g

DIRECTIONS

1. In the mixing bowl, mix up together grated zucchini, diced onion, eggs, coconut flour, salt, ground black pepper, crumbled cheese, chopped spinach, baking powder, and lemon juice.

2. Add butter and churn the mixture until homogenous.

3. Line the baking dish with baking paper.

4. Transfer the zucchini mixture into the baking dish and flatten it.

5. Preheat the oven to 365F and put the dish inside.

6. Cook it for 15 minutes. Then chill the meal well.

7. Cut it into bars.

MUSHROOM SOUP

PREPARATION
10 MINS

COOKING
25 MINS

SERVINGS
4

INGREDIENTS

- 1 cup of water
- 1 cup of coconut milk
- 1 cup white mushrooms, chopped
- ½ carrot, chopped
- ¼ white onion, diced
- 1 tablespoon butter

- 2 oz turnip, chopped
- 1 teaspoon dried dill
- ½ teaspoon ground black pepper
- ¾ teaspoon smoked paprika
- 1 oz celery stalk, chopped

NUTRIRION

- Calories: 39
- Total Fat: 2.6 g
- Cholesterol: 0 mg
- Sodium: 340 mg

- Potassium: 31 mg
- Total Carbohydrate: 3.3 g
- Protein: 0.7 g

DIRECTIONS

1. Pour water and coconut milk in the saucepan. Bring the liquid to boil.

2. Add chopped mushrooms, carrot, and turnip. Close the lid and boil for 10 minutes.

3. Meanwhile, put butter in the skillet. Add diced onion. Sprinkle it with dill, ground black pepper, and smoked paprika. Roast the onion for 3 minutes.

4. Add the roasted onion in the soup mixture.

5. Then add chopped celery stalk. Close the lid.

6. Cook soup for 10 minutes.

7. Then ladle it into the serving bowls.

STUFFED PORTOBELLO MUSHROOMS

PREPARATION
10 MINS

COOKING
10 MINS

SERVINGS
4

INGREDIENTS

- 2 portobello mushrooms
- 1 cup spinach, chopped, steamed
- 2 oz artichoke hearts, drained, chopped
- 1 tablespoon coconut cream
- 1 tablespoon cream cheese
- 1 teaspoon minced garlic

- 1 tablespoon fresh cilantro, chopped
- 3 oz Cheddar cheese, grated
- ½ teaspoon ground black pepper
- 2 tablespoons olive oil
- ½ teaspoon salt

NUTRIRION

- Calories: 135.2
- Total Fat: 5.5 g
- Cholesterol: 16.4 mg
- Sodium : 698.1 mg

- Potassium: 275.3 mg
- Total Carbohydrate: 8.4 g
- Protein: 14.8 g

DIRECTIONS

1. Sprinkle mushrooms with olive oil and place in the tray.

2. Transfer the tray in the preheated to 360F oven and broil them for 5 minutes.

3. Meanwhile, blend artichoke hearts, coconut cream, cream cheese, minced garlic, and chopped cilantro.

4. Add grated cheese in the mixture and sprinkle with ground black pepper and salt.

5. Fill the broiled mushrooms with the cheese mixture and cook them for 5 minutes more. Serve the mushrooms only hot

Lettuce Salad

PREPARATION
10 MINS

COOKING
0 MINS

SERVINGS
1

INGREDIENTS

- 1 cup Romaine lettuce, roughly chopped

- 3 oz seitan, chopped

- 1 tablespoon avocado oil

- 1 teaspoon sunflower seeds

- 1 teaspoon lemon juice

- 1 egg, boiled, peeled

- 2 oz Cheddar cheese, shredded

NUTRIRION

- Calories 20

- Total Fat 0.2g

- Cholesterol 0mg

- Sodium 31mg

- Potassium 241mg

- Total Carbohydrates 4.2g

- Protein 1.2g

DIRECTIONS

1. Place lettuce in the salad bowl. Add chopped seitan and shredded cheese.

2. Then chop the egg roughly and add in the salad bowl too.

3. Mix up together lemon juice with the avocado oil.

4. Sprinkle the salad with the oil mixture and sunflower seeds. Don't stir the salad before serving.

ONION SOUP

PREPARATION
10 MINS

COOKING
25 MINS

SERVINGS
6

INGREDIENTS

- 2 cups white onion, diced

- 4 tablespoon butter

- ½ cup white mushrooms, chopped

- 3 cups of water

- 1 cup heavy cream

- 1 teaspoon salt

- 1 teaspoon chili flakes

- 1 teaspoon garlic powder

NUTRIRION

- Calories: 290.

- Fat: 9.6g.

- Protein: 16.8g.

- Carbohydrate: 33.4g.

DIRECTIONS

1. PPut butter in the saucepan and melt it.

2. Add diced white onion, chili flakes, and garlic powder. Mix it up and saute for 10 minutes over the medium-low heat.

3. Then add water, heavy cream, and chopped mushrooms. Close the lid.

4. Cook the soup for 15 minutes more.

5. Then blend the soup until you get the creamy texture. Ladle it in the bowls.

ASPARAGUS SALAD

PREPARATION
10 MINS

COOKING
15 MINS

SERVINGS
3

INGREDIENTS

- 10 oz asparagus

- 1 tablespoon olive oil

- ½ teaspoon white pepper

- 4 oz Feta cheese, crumbled

- 1 cup lettuce, chopped

- 1 tablespoon canola oil

- 1 teaspoon apple cider vinegar

- 1 tomato, diced

NUTRIRION

- Calories: 87.5

- Total Fat: 4.1 g

- Cholesterol: 9.2 mg

- Sodium: 685.8 mg

- Potassium: 212.1 mg

- Total Carbohydrate: 8.1 g

- Protein: 5.1 g

DIRECTIONS

1. SPreheat the oven to 365F.

2. Place asparagus in the tray, sprinkle with olive oil and white pepper and transfer in the preheated oven. Cook it for 15 minutes.

3. Meanwhile, put crumbled Feta in the salad bowl.

4. Add chopped lettuce and diced tomato.

5. Sprinkle the ingredients with apple cider vinegar.

6. Chill the cooked asparagus to the room temperature and add in the salad.

7. Shake the salad gently before serving.

BEEF WITH CABBAGE NOODLES

PREPARATION
5 MINS

COOKING
18 MINS

SERVINGS
2

INGREDIENTS

- 4 oz ground beef
- 1 cup chopped cabbage
- 4 oz tomato sauce
- ½ tsp minced garlic
- ½ cup of water
- Seasoning:

- ½ tbsp coconut oil
- ½ tsp salt
- ¼ tsp Italian seasoning
- 1/8 tsp dried basil

NUTRIRION

- Calories: 188.5
- Fats: 12.5 g
- Protein: 15.5 g

- Net Carbohydrates: 2.5 g
- Fiber: 1 g

DIRECTIONS

1. Take a skillet pan, place it over medium heat, add oil and when hot, add beef and cook for 5 minutes until nicely browned.

2. Meanwhile, prepare the cabbage and, for it, slice the cabbage into thin shred.

3. When the beef has cooked, add garlic, season with salt, basil, and Italian seasoning, stir well and continue cooking for 3 minutes until beef has thoroughly cooked.

4. Pour in tomato sauce and water, stir well and bring the mixture to boil.

5. Then reduce heat to medium-low level, add cabbage, stir well until well mixed and simmer for 3 to 5 minutes until cabbage is softened, covering the pan.

6. Uncover the pan and continue simmering the beef until most of the cooking liquid has evaporated.

7. Serve.

ROAST BEEF AND MOZZARELLA PLATE

PREPARATION
5 MINS

COOKING
0 MINS

SERVINGS
2

INGREDIENTS

- 4 slices of roast beef
- ½ ounce chopped lettuce
- 1 avocado, pitted
- 2 oz mozzarella cheese, cubed
- ½ cup mayonnaise

- Seasoning:
- ¼ tsp salt
- 1/8 tsp ground black pepper
- 2 tbsp avocado oil

NUTRIRION

- Calories: 267.7
- Fats: 24.5 g
- Protein: 9.5 g

- Net Carbohydrates: 1.5 g
- Fiber: 2 g

DIRECTIONS

1. Scoop out flesh from avocado and divide it evenly between two plates.

2. Add slices of roast beef, lettuce, and cheese and then sprinkle with salt and black pepper.

3. Serve with avocado oil and mayonnaise.

BEEF AND BROCCOLI

PREPARATION
5 MINS

COOKING
10 MINS

SERVINGS
2

INGREDIENTS

- 6 slices of beef roast, cut into strips
- 1 scallion, chopped
- 3 oz broccoli florets, chopped
- 1 tbsp avocado oil
- 1 tbsp butter, unsalted

- Seasoning:
- ¼ tsp salt
- 1/8 tsp ground black pepper
- 1 ½ tbsp soy sauce
- 3 tbsp chicken broth

NUTRIRION

- Calories: 15.7 g
- Fats: 21.6 g

- Protein: 1.7 g
- Net Carbohydrates:1.3 g

DIRECTIONS

1. Take a medium skillet pan, place it over medium heat, add oil and when hot, add beef strips and cook for 2 minutes until hot.

2. Transfer beef to a plate, add scallion to the pan, then add butter and cook for 3 minutes until tender.

3. Add remaining ingredients, stir until mixed, switch heat to the low level, and simmer for 3 to 4 minutes until broccoli is tender.

4. Return beef to the pan, stir until well combined and cook for 1 minute.

5. Serve

GARLIC HERB BEEF ROAST

PREPARATION
5 MINS

COOKING
10 MINS

SERVINGS
2

INGREDIENTS

- 6 slices of beef roast

- ½ tsp garlic powder

- 1/3 tsp dried thyme

- ¼ tsp dried rosemary

- 2 tbsp butter, unsalted

- Seasoning:

- 1/3 tsp salt

- 1/4 tsp ground black pepper

NUTRIRION

- Calories: 140

- Fats: 12.7 g

- Protein: 5.5 g

- Net Carbohydrates: 0.1 g

- Fiber: 0.2 g

DIRECTIONS

1. Prepare the spice mix and for this, take a small bowl, place garlic powder, thyme, rosemary, salt, and black pepper and then stir until mixed.

2. Sprinkle spice mix on the beef roast.

3. Take a medium skillet pan, place it over medium heat, add butter and when it melts, add beef roast and then cook for 5 to 8 minutes until golden brown and cooked.

4. Serve.

Sprouts Stir-fry with Kale, Broccoli, and Beef

PREPARATION
5 MINS

COOKING
8 MINS

SERVINGS
2

INGREDIENTS

- 3 slices of beef roast, chopped
- 2 oz Brussels sprouts, halved
- 4 oz broccoli florets
- 3 oz kale
- 1 ½ tbsp butter, unsalted

- 1/8 tsp red pepper flakes
- Seasoning:
- ¼ tsp garlic powder
- ¼ tsp salt
- 1/8 tsp ground black pepper

NUTRIRION

- Calories: 140
- Fats: 12.7 g
- Protein: 5.5 g

- Net Carbohydrates: 0.1 g
- Fiber: 0.2 g

DIRECTIONS

1. Take a medium skillet pan, place it over medium heat, add ¾ tbsp butter and when it melts, add broccoli florets and sprouts, sprinkle with garlic powder, and cook for 2 minutes.

2. Season vegetables with salt and red pepper flakes, add chopped beef, stir until mixed and continue cooking for 3 minutes until browned on one side.

3. Then add kale along with remaining butter, flip the vegetables and cook for 2 minutes until kale leaves wilts.

4. Serve.

BEEF AND VEGETABLE SKILLET

PREPARATION
5 MINS

COOKING
15 MINS

SERVINGS
2

INGREDIENTS

- 3 oz spinach, chopped
- ½ pound ground beef
- 2 slices of bacon, diced
- 2 oz chopped asparagus
- Seasoning:

- 3 tbsp coconut oil
- 2 tsp dried thyme
- 2/3 tsp salt
- ½ tsp ground black pepper

NUTRIRION

- Calories 332.5
- Fats 26 g;
- Protein 23.5 g;

- Carbohydrates 1.5 g
- Fiber 1 g

DIRECTIONS

1. Take a skillet pan, place it over medium heat, add oil and when hot, add beef and bacon and cook for 5 to 7 minutes until slightly browned.

2. Then add asparagus and spinach, sprinkle with thyme, stir well and cook for 7 to 10 minutes until thoroughly cooked.

3. Season skillet with salt and black pepper and serve.

BEEF, PEPPER AND GREEN BEANS STIR-FRY

PREPARATION
5 MINS

COOKING
18 MINS

SERVINGS
2

INGREDIENTS

- 6 oz ground beef

- 2 oz chopped green bell pepper

- 4 oz green beans

- 3 tbsp grated cheddar cheese

- Seasoning:

- ½ tsp salt

- ¼ tsp ground black pepper

- ¼ tsp paprika

NUTRIRION

- Calories: 282.5

- Fats: 17.6 g

- Protein: 26.1 g

- Net Carbohydrates: 2.9 g

DIRECTIONS

1. Take a skillet pan, place it over medium heat, add ground beef and cook for 4 minutes until slightly browned.

2. Then add bell pepper and green beans, season with salt, paprika, and black pepper, stir well and continue cooking for 7 to 10 minutes until beef and vegetables have cooked through.

3. Sprinkle cheddar cheese on top, then transfer pan under the broiler and cook for 2 minutes until cheese has melted and the top is golden brown. And serve

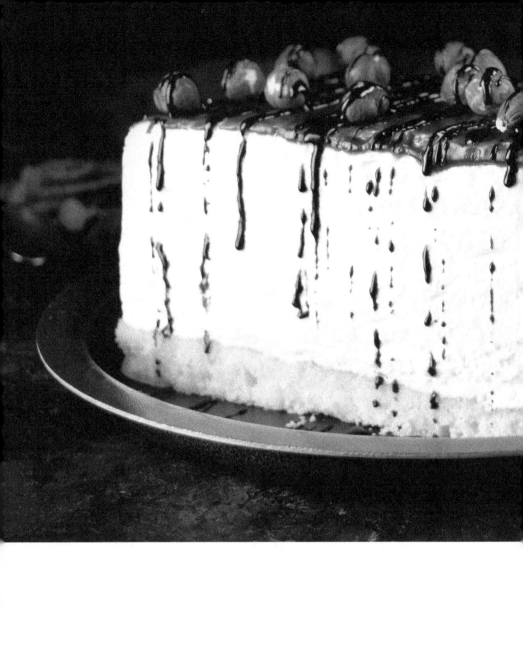

CHAPTER 09

DESSERT

KETO CHEESECAKES

PREPARATION
25 MINS

SERVINGS
6

INGREDIENTS

- **FOR THE CHEESECAKES:**

- 2 tablespoons butter

- 1 tablespoon caramel syrup; sugar-free

- 3 tablespoons coffee

- 8 ounces cream cheese

- 1/3 cup swerve sweetener

- 3 eggs

- **FOR THE FROSTING:**

- 8 ounces mascarpone cheese; soft

- 3 tablespoons caramel syrup; sugar-free

- 2 tablespoons swerve

- 3 tablespoons butter

NUTRIRION

- Calories: 478.2

- Total Fat: 47.8 g

- Cholesterol: 140.4 mg

- Sodium : 270.7 mg

- Potassium: 233.7 mg

- Total Carbohydrate: 9.4 g

- Protein: 9.2 g

DIRECTIONS

1. In your blender, mix cream cheese with eggs, 2 tablespoons butter, coffee, 1 tablespoon caramel syrup, and 1/3 cup swerve. Pulse very well.

2. Spoon this into a cupcakes pan, introduce in the oven at 350 degrees F and bake for 15 minutes

3. Leave aside to cool down and then keep in the freezer for 3 hours

4. Meanwhile, in a bowl, mix 3 tablespoons butter with 3 tablespoons caramel syrup, 2 tablespoons swerve, and mascarpone cheese and blend well.

5. Spoon this over cheesecakes and serve them.

KETO BROWNIES

PREPARATION
30 MINS

SERVINGS
12

INGREDIENTS

- 6 ounces coconut oil; melted
- 4 ounces cream cheese
- 5 tablespoons swerve sweetener
- 6 eggs

- 2 teaspoons vanilla
- 3 ounces of cocoa powder
- 1/2 teaspoon baking powder

NUTRIRION

- Calories: 183.7
- Total Fat: 16.6 g
- Cholesterol: 20.7 mg
- Sodium : 36.3 mg

- Potassium: 21.6 mg
- Total Carbohydrate: 4.9 g
- Protein: 1.4 g

DIRECTIONS

1. In a blender, mix eggs with coconut oil, cocoa powder, baking powder, vanilla, cream cheese, and swerve. Stir using a mixer.

2. Pour this into a lined baking dish, introduce in the oven at 350 degrees F and bake for 20 minutes

3. Slice into rectangle pieces when it gets cold and serve

RASPBERRY AND COCONUT

PREPARATION
15 MINS

SERVINGS
12

INGREDIENTS

- 1/4 cup swerve sweetener

- 1/2 cup coconut oil

- 1/2 cup raspberries; dried

- 1/2 cup coconut; shredded

- 1/2 cup coconut butter

NUTRIRION

- Carbohydrates: 45g

- Sugar: 30g

- Fat: 42g

- Protein: 8g

- Cholesterol: 0mg

DIRECTIONS

1. In your food processor, blend dried berries very well.

2. Heat a pan with the butter over medium heat.

3. Add oil, coconut and swerve; stir and cook for 5 minutes

4. Pour half of this into a lined baking pan and spread well.

5. Add raspberry powder and also spread.

6. Top with the rest of the butter mix, spread and keep in the fridge for a while

7. Cut into pieces and serve

Chocolate Pudding Delight

PREPARATION
52 MINS

SERVINGS
2

INGREDIENTS

- 1/2 teaspoon stevia powder
- 2 tablespoons cocoa powder
- 2 tablespoons water
- 1 tablespoon gelatin
- 1 cup of coconut milk
- 2 tablespoons maple syrup

NUTRIRION

- Calories: 221.2
- Total Fat: 13.6 g
- Cholesterol: 9.8 mg
- Sodium : 250.3 mg
- Potassium: 86.7 mg
- Total Carbohydrate: 22.7 g
- Protein: 3.4 g

DIRECTIONS

1. Heat a pan with the coconut milk over medium heat; add stevia and cocoa powder and mix well.

2. In a bowl, mix gelatin with water; stir well and add to the pan.

3. Stir well, add maple syrup, whisk again, divide into ramekins and keep in the fridge for 45 minutes Serve cold.

PEANUT BUTTER FUDGE

PREPARATION
132 MINS

SERVINGS
12

INGREDIENTS

- 1 cup peanut butter; unsweetened

- 1 cup of coconut oil

- 1/4 cup almond milk

- 2 teaspoons vanilla stevia

- A pinch of salt

- For the topping:

- 2 tablespoons swerve sweetener

- 1/4 cup cocoa powder

- 2 tablespoons melted coconut oil

NUTRIRION

- Calories: 85

- Fat: 4.7g

- Saturated Fat: 2.7g

- Protein: 0.5g

DIRECTIONS

1. In a heatproof bowl, mix peanut butter with 1 cup coconut oil; stir and heat up in your microwave until it melts

2. Add a pinch of salt, almond milk, and stevia; stir well everything and pour into a lined loaf pan.

3. Keep in the fridge for 2 hours and then slice it.

4. In a bowl, mix 2 tablespoons melted coconut with cocoa powder and swerve and stir very well.

5. Drizzle the sauce over your peanut butter fudge and serve

CINNAMON STREUSEL EGG LOAF

PREPARATION
10 MINS

COOKING
15 MINS

SERVINGS
2

INGREDIENTS

- 2 tbsp almond flour
- 1 tbsp butter, softened
- ½ tbsp grated butter, chilled
- 1 egg
- 1-ounce cream cheese

- Others:
- ½ tsp cinnamon, divided
- 1 tbsp erythritol sweetener, divided
- ¼ tsp vanilla extract, unsweetened

NUTRIRION

- Calories: 152
- Fats: 14.8 g
- Protein: 4.1 g

- Net Carbohydrates: 1.3 g
- Fiber: 0.9 g

DIRECTIONS

1. Turn on the oven, then set it to 350 degrees F and let it preheat.

2. Meanwhile, crack the egg in a small bowl, add cream cheese, softened butter, ¼ tsp cinnamon, ½ tbsp sweetener, and vanilla and whisk until well combined.

3. Divide the egg batter between two silicone muffins and then bake for 7 minutes.

4. Meanwhile, prepare the streusel and for this, place flour in a small bowl, add remaining ingredients and stir until well mixed.

5. When egg loaves have baked, sprinkle streusel on top and then continue baking for 7 minutes.

6. When done, remove loaves from the cups, let them cool for 5 minutes and then serve and enjoy!

Snickerdoodle Muffins

PREPARATION
10 MINS

COOKING
12 MINS

SERVINGS
2

INGREDIENTS

- 6 2/3 tbsp coconut flour

- ½ of egg

- 1 tbsp butter, unsalted, melted

- 1 1/3 tbsp whipping cream

- 1 tbsp almond milk, unsweetened

- Others:

- 1 1/3 tbsp erythritol sweetener and more for topping

- ¼ tsp baking powder

- ¼ tsp ground cinnamon and more for topping

- ¼ tsp vanilla extract, unsweetened

NUTRIRION

- Calories: 241

- Fats: 21 g

- Protein: 7 g

- Net Carbohydrates: 3 g

- Fiber: 3 g

DIRECTIONS

1. Turn on the oven, then set it to 350 degrees F and let it preheat.

2. Meanwhile, take a medium bowl, place flour in it, add cinnamon and baking powder. Stir until combined.

3. Take a separate bowl, place the half egg in it, add butter, sour cream, milk, and vanilla and whisk until blended.

4. Whisk in flour mixture until a smooth batter is obtained, divide the batter evenly between two silicon muffin cups and then sprinkle cinnamon and sweetener on top.

5. Bake the muffins for 10 to 12 minutes until firm, and then the top has turned golden brown and then serve and enjoy!

Yogurt and Strawberry Bowl

PREPARATION
5 MINS

COOKING
0 MINS

SERVINGS
2

INGREDIENTS

- 3 oz mixed berries
- 1 tbsp chopped almonds
- 1 tbsp chopped walnuts
- 4 oz yogurt

DIRECTIONS

1. Divide yogurt between two bowls, top with berries and then sprinkle with almonds and walnuts.

2. Serve and enjoy!

NUTRIRION

- Calories: 165
- Fats: 11.2 g
- Protein: 9.3 g
- Net Carbohydrates: 2.5 g
- Fiber: 1.8 g

Sweet Cinnamon Muffin

PREPARATION
5 MINS

COOKING
2 MINS

SERVINGS
2

INGREDIENTS

- 4 tsp coconut flour
- 2 tsp cinnamon
- 2 tsp erythritol sweetener
- 1/16 tsp baking soda
- 2 eggs

DIRECTIONS

1. Take a medium bowl, place all the ingredients in it, and whisk until well combined.

2. Take two ramekins, grease them with oil, distribute the prepared batter in it and then microwave for 1 minute and 45 seconds until done.

3. When done, take out muffin from the ramekin, cut in half, and then serve and enjoy

NUTRIRION

- Calories: 101
- Fats: 6.5 g
- Protein: 7.6 g
- Net Carbohydrates: 0.5 g
- Fiber: 1.7 g

Nutty Muffins

PREPARATION
5 MINS

COOKING
5 MINS

SERVINGS
2

INGREDIENTS

- 4 tsp coconut flour
- 1/16 tsp baking soda
- 1 tsp erythritol sweetener
- 2 eggs
- 2 tsp almond butter, unsalted

NUTRIRION

- Calories: 131
- Fats: 8.6 g
- Protein: 8.4 g
- Net Carbohydrates: 2.3 g
- Fiber: 2.2 g

DIRECTIONS

1. Take a medium bowl, place all the ingredients in it, and whisk until well combined.

2. Take two ramekins, grease them with oil, distribute the prepared batter in it and then microwave for 1 minute and 45 seconds until done.

3. When done, take out muffin from the ramekin, cut in half, and then serve and enjoy!

Pumpkin and Cream Cheese Cup

PREPARATION
10 MINS

COOKING
12 MINS

SERVINGS
2

INGREDIENTS

- 4 tbsp almond flour

- 1 1/3 tbsp coconut flour

- 2 tbsp pumpkin puree

- 2 2/3 tbsp cream cheese, softened

- ½ of egg

- 2/3 tbsp butter, unsalted

- ¼ tsp pumpkin spice

- 2/3 tsp baking powder

- 2 tbsp erythritol sweetener

NUTRIRION

- Calories: 261

- Fats: 23 g

- Protein: 7 g

- Net Carbohydrates: 2 g

- Fiber: 4 g

DIRECTIONS

1. Turn on the oven, then set it to 350 degrees F and let it preheat.

2. Take a medium bowl, place butter and 1 ½ tbsp sweetener in it, and then beat until fluffy.

3. Beat in egg and then beat in pumpkin puree until well combined.

4. Take a medium bowl, place flours in it, stir in pumpkin spice, baking powder until mixed, stir this mixture into the butter mixture and then distribute it into two silicone muffin cups.

5. Take a medium bowl, place cream cheese in it, and stir in remaining sweetener until well combined.

6. Divide the cream cheese mixture into the silicone muffin cups, swirl the batter and cream cheese mixture by using a toothpick and then bake for 10 to 12 minutes until muffins have turned firm.

7. Serve and enjoy!

BERRIES IN YOGURT CREAM

PREPARATION
65 MINS

COOKING
0 MINS

SERVINGS
2

INGREDIENTS

- 1-ounce blackberries
- 1-ounce raspberry
- 2 tbsp erythritol sweetener
- 4 oz yogurt
- 4 oz whipping cream

NUTRIRION

- Calories: 245
- Fats: 22 g
- Protein: 4.2 g
- Net Carbohydrates: 5 g
- Fiber: 1.7

DIRECTIONS

1. Take a medium bowl, place yogurt in it, and then whisk in cream.

2. Sprinkle sweetener over yogurt mixture, don't stir, cover the bowl with a lid, and then refrigerate for 1 hour.

3. When ready to serve, stir the yogurt mixture, divide it evenly between two bowls, top with berries, and then serve and enjoy!

PUMPKIN PIE MUG CAKE

PREPARATION
5 MINS

COOKING
2 MINS

SERVINGS
2

INGREDIENTS

- 2 tbsp coconut flour
- 1 tsp sour cream
- 2 tbsp whipping cream
- 2 eggs
- ¼ cup pumpkin puree

- Others:
- 2 tbsp erythritol sweetener
- 1/3 tsp cinnamon
- ¼ tsp baking soda

NUTRIRION

- Calories: 245
- Fats: 22 g
- Protein: 4.2 g

- Net Carbohydrates: 5 g
- Fiber: 1.7

DIRECTIONS

1. Take a small bowl, place cream in it, and then beat in sweetener until well combined.

2. Cover the bowl, let it chill in the refrigerator for 30 minutes, then beat in eggs and pumpkin puree and stir in remaining ingredients until incorporated and smooth.

3. Divide the batter between two coffee mugs greased with oil and then microwave for 2 minutes until thoroughly cooked.

4. Serve and enjoy!

CHOCOLATE AND STRAWBERRY CREPE

PREPARATION
5 MINS

COOKING
5 MINS

SERVINGS
2

INGREDIENTS

- 1 1/3 tbsp coconut flour

- 1 tsp of cocoa powder

- ¼ tsp flaxseed

- 1 egg

- 2 ¾ tbsp coconut milk, unsweetened

- 2 tsp avocado oil

- 1/8 tsp baking powder

- 2 oz strawberry, sliced

NUTRIRION

- Calories 120

- Fats 8.5 g

- Protein 4.4 g

- Carbohydrates 2.8 g

- Fiber 2.7 g

DIRECTIONS

1. Take a medium bowl, place flour in it, and then stir in cocoa powder, baking powder, and flaxseed in it until mixed.

2. Add egg and milk and then whisk until smooth.

3. Take a medium skillet pan, place it over medium heat, add 1 tsp oil and when hot, pour in half of the batter, spread it evenly, and then cook for 1 minute per side until firm.

4. Transfer crepe to a plate, add remaining oil, and cook another crepe by using the remaining batter.

5. When done, fill crepes with strawberries, fold them and then serve and enjoy

BLACKBERRY AND COCONUT FLOUR CUPCAKE

PREPARATION
5 MINS

COOKING
15 MINS

SERVINGS
2

INGREDIENTS

- 3 ¼ tbsp coconut flour

- 1/3 cup whipping cream

- 1 tbsp cream cheese

- 1 ½ egg

- 1-ounce blackberry

- 2 2/3 tbsp butter, unsalted,

- chopped

- 5 1/3 tbsp erythritol sweetener

- 2/3 tsp baking powder

- 1/3 tsp vanilla extract, unsweetened

NUTRIRION

- Calorie: 420

- Fats: 38.2 g

- Protein: 9.4 g

- Net Carbohydrates: 5.7 g

- Fiber: 4.8 g

DIRECTIONS

1. Take a small bowl, place butter in it, add cream and them microwave for 30 to 60 seconds until it melts, stirring every 20 seconds.

2. Then add cream cheese, cream, vanilla, and erythritol, whisk until smooth, whisk in coconut flour and baking powder until incorporated and then fold in berries.

3. Distribute the mixture evenly between four muffin cups, then bake for 12 to 15 minutes until firm.

4. Serve and enjoy!

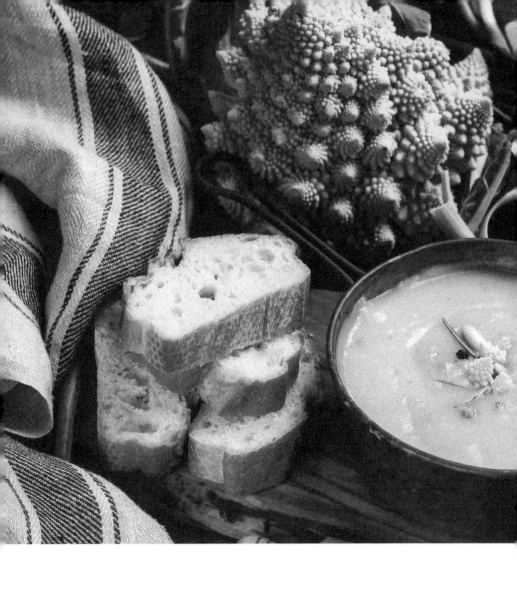

CHAPTER 10

SOUP

Coconut Soup

PREPARATION
12 MINS

COOKING
35 MINS

SERVINGS
4

INGREDIENTS

- 2 cloves garlic

- 1 medium white onion

- 1 tbsp butter

- 2 cups of water

- 2 cups vegetable stock

- 1 cup heavy cream

- Salt and ground black pepper to taste

- ½ tsp paprika

- 1½ cups broccoli, divided into florets

- 1 cup cheddar cheese

NUTRIRION

- Calories: 348

- Carbohydrates: 6.8g

- Fat: 33.8g

- Protein: 10.9g

DIRECTIONS

1. Peel and mince garlic. Peel and chop the onion.

2. Preheat pot on medium heat, add butter and melt it.

3. Add garlic and onion and sauté for 5 minutes, stirring occasionally.

4. Pour in water, vegetable stock, heavy cream, and add pepper, salt, and paprika.

5. Stir and bring to boil.

6. Add broccoli and simmer for 25 minutes.

7. After that, transfer soup mixture to a food processor and blend well.

8. Grate cheddar cheese and add to a food processor, blend again.

9. Serve soup hot.

Broccoli Soup

PREPARATION
12 MINS

COOKING
35 MINS

SERVINGS
4

INGREDIENTS

- 2 cloves garlic

- 1 medium white onion

- 1 tbsp butter

- 2 cups of water

- 2 cups vegetable stock

- 1 cup heavy cream

- Salt and ground black pepper to taste

- ½ tsp paprika

- 1½ cups broccoli, divided into florets

- 1 cup cheddar cheese

NUTRIRION

- Calories: 348

- Carbohydrates: 6.8g

- Fat: 33.8g

- Protein: 10.9g

DIRECTIONS

1. Peel and mince garlic. Peel and chop the onion.

2. Preheat pot on medium heat, add butter and melt it.

3. Add garlic and onion and sauté for 5 minutes, stirring occasionally.

4. Pour in water, vegetable stock, heavy cream, and add pepper, salt, and paprika.

5. Stir and bring to boil.

6. Add broccoli and simmer for 25 minutes.

7. After that, transfer soup mixture to a food processor and blend well.

8. Grate cheddar cheese and add to a food processor, blend again.

9. Serve soup hot.

SIMPLE TOMATO SOUP

PREPARATION
15 MINS

COOKING
10 MINS

SERVINGS
6

INGREDIENTS

- 4 cups canned tomato soup

- 2 tbsp apple cider vinegar

- 1 tsp dried oregano

- 4 tbsp butter

- 2 tsp turmeric

- 2 oz red hot sauce

- Salt and ground black pepper to taste

- 4 tbsp olive oil

- 8 bacon strips, cooked and crumbled

- 4 oz fresh basil leaves, chopped

- 4 oz green onions, chopped

NUTRIRION

- Calories: 397

- Carbohydrates: 9.8g

- Fat: 33.8

- Protein: 11.7g

DIRECTIONS

1. Pour tomato soup in the pot and preheat on medium heat. Bring to boil.

2. Add vinegar, oregano, butter, turmeric, hot sauce, salt, black pepper, and olive oil. Stir well.

3. Simmer the soup for 5 minutes.

4. Serve soup topped with crumbled bacon, green onion, and basil.

GREEN SOUP

PREPARATION
12 MINS

COOKING
15 MINS

SERVINGS
6

INGREDIENTS

- 2 cloves garlic
- 1 white onion
- 1 cauliflower head
- 2 oz butter
- 1 bay leaf, crushed
- 1 cup spinach leaves

- ½ cup watercress
- 4 cups vegetable stock
- Salt and ground black pepper to taste
- 1 cup of coconut milk
- ½ cup parsley, for serving

NUTRIRION

- Calories: 227
- Carbohydrates: 4.89g

- Fat: 35.1
- Protein: 6.97g

DIRECTIONS

1. Peel and mince garlic. Peel and dice onion.

2. Divide cauliflower into florets.

3. Preheat pot on medium-high heat, add butter and melt it.

4. Add onion and garlic, stir, and sauté for 4 minutes.

5. Add cauliflower and bay leaf, stir and cook for 5 minutes.

6. Add spinach and watercress, stir and cook for another 3 minutes.

7. Pour in vegetable stock—season with salt and black pepper. Stir and bring to boil.

8. Pour in coconut milk and stir well. Take off heat.

9. Use an immersion blender to blend well.

10. Top with parsley and serve hot.

SAUSAGE AND PEPPERS SOUP

PREPARATION
15 MINS

COOKING
75 MINS

SERVINGS
6

INGREDIENTS

- 1 tbsp avocado oil

- 2 lbs pork sausage meat

- Salt and ground black pepper to taste

- 1 green bell pepper, seeded and chopped

- 5 oz canned jalapeños, chopped

- 5 oz canned tomatoes, chopped

- 1¼ cup spinach

- 4 cups beef stock

- 1 tsp Italian seasoning

- 1 tbsp cumin

- 1 tsp onion powder

- 1 tsp garlic powder

- 1 tbsp chili powder

NUTRIRION

- Calories: 227

- Carbohydrates: 4.89g

- Fat: 35.1

- Protein: 6.97g

DIRECTIONS

1. Preheat pot with avocado oil on medium heat.

2. Put sausage meat in pot and brown for 3 minutes on all sides.

3. Add salt, black pepper, and green bell pepper and continue to cook for 3 minutes.

4. Add jalapeños and tomatoes, stir well and cook for 2 minutes more.

5. Toss spinach and stir again close lid and cook for 7 minutes.

6. Pour in beef stock, Italian seasoning, cumin, onion powder, chili powder, garlic powder, salt, and black pepper, stir well. Close lid again. Cook for 30 minutes.

7. When time is up, uncover the pot and simmer for 15 minutes more.

8. Serve hot.

Avocado Soup

PREPARATION
12 MINS

COOKING
15 MINS

SERVINGS
4

INGREDIENTS

- 2 tbsp butter
- 2 scallions, chopped
- 3 cups chicken stock
- 2 avocados, pitted, peeled, and chopped
- Salt and ground black pepper to taste
- ⅔ cup heavy cream

NUTRIRION

- Calories: 329
- Carbohydrates: 5.9g
- Fat: 22.9g
- Protein: 5.8g

DIRECTIONS

1. Preheat pot on medium heat, add butter and melt it.

2. Toss scallions, stir and sauté for 2 minutes.

3. Pour in 2 ½ cups stock and bring to simmer—Cook for 3 minutes.

4. Meanwhile, peel and chop avocados.

5. Place avocado, ½ cup of stock, cream, salt, and pepper in a blender and blend well.

6. Add avocado mixture to the pot and mix well—Cook for 2 minutes.

7. Sprinkle with more salt and pepper, stir.

8. Serve hot.

Avocado and Bacon Soup

PREPARATION
15 MINS

COOKING
15 MINS

SERVINGS
6

INGREDIENTS

- 1-quart chicken stock

- 2 avocados, pitted

- ⅓ cup fresh cilantro, chopped

- 1 tsp garlic powder

- Salt and ground black pepper to taste

- Juice of ½ lime

- ½ lb bacon, cooked and chopped

NUTRIRION

- Calories: 298

- Carbohydrates: 5.98g

- Fat: 22.8g

- Protein: 16.8g

DIRECTIONS

1. Pour chicken stock in a pot and bring to boil over medium-high heat.

2. Meanwhile, peel and chop the avocados.

3. Place avocados, cilantro, garlic powder, salt, black pepper, and lime juice in blender or food processor and blend well.

4. Add the avocado mixture in boiling stock and stir well.

5. Add bacon and season with salt and pepper to taste.

6. Stir and simmer for 3-4 minutes on medium heat.

7. Serve hot.

ROASTED BELL PEPPERS SOUP

PREPARATION
15 MINS

COOKING
20 MINS

SERVINGS
6

INGREDIENTS

- 1 medium white onion

- 2 cloves garlic

- 2 celery stalks

- 12 oz roasted bell peppers, seeded

- 2 tbsp olive oil

- Salt and ground black pepper

to taste

- 1-quart chicken stock

- 2/3 cup water

- ¼ cup Parmesan cheese, grated

- ⅔ cup heavy cream

NUTRIRION

- Calories: 180

- Carbohydrates: 3.9g

- Fat: 12.9g

- Protein: 5.9g

DIRECTIONS

1. Directions:

2. Peel and chop onion and garlic. Chop celery and bell pepper.

3. Preheat pot with oil on medium heat.

4. Put garlic, onion, celery, salt, and pepper in the pot, stir and sauté for 8 minutes.

5. Pour in chicken stock and water. Add bell peppers and stir.

6. Bring to boil, close lid, and simmer for 5 minutes. Reduce heat if needed.

7. When time is up, blend soup using an immersion blender.

8. Add cream and season with salt and pepper to taste. Take off heat.

9. Serve hot with grated cheese.

SPICY BACON SOUP

PREPARATION
15 MINS

COOKING
30 MINS

SERVINGS
6

INGREDIENTS

- 10 oz bacon, chopped

- Salt to taste

- 1 tbsp olive oil

- 2/3 cup cauliflower, divided into florets

- 4 oz green bell pepper, seeded and chopped

- 1 jalapeno pepper, seeded and chopped

- 4 cups chicken stock

- 2 tbsp full-fat cream

- 1 tsp ground black pepper

- 1 tsp chili pepper

NUTRIRION

- Calories: 301

- Carbohydrates: 3.9g

- Fat: 23g

- Protein: 19g

DIRECTIONS

1. In a bowl, combine bacon with salt.

2. Heat a pan over medium heat and cook bacon for 5 minutes, stirring constantly.

3. Remove bacon from pan and set aside.

4. Pour olive oil in a pan and add cauliflower, bell pepper, and jalapeno.

5. Cook veggies on high heat for 1 minute, stirring occasionally.

6. In a saucepan, mix bacon with vegetables. Pour in chicken stock. Stir.

7. Close lid and cook for 20-25 minutes.

8. Open the lid and add cream, stir.

9. Season with salt, black pepper, and chili pepper. Stir and cook for 5 minutes more.

10.   Serve.

ITALIAN SAUSAGE SOUP

PREPARATION
15 MINS

COOKING
35 MINS

SERVINGS
10

INGREDIENTS

- 1 tsp avocado oil
- 2 cloves garlic
- 1 medium white onion
- 1½ lbs hot pork sausage, chopped
- 8 cups chicken stock
- 1 lb radishes, chopped

- 10 oz spinach
- 1 cup heavy cream
- 6 bacon slices, chopped
- Salt and ground black pepper to taste
- A pinch of red pepper flakes

NUTRIRION

- Calories: 289
- Carbohydrates: 3.8g

- Fat: 21.8g
- Protein: 18.1g

DIRECTIONS

1. Preheat pot on medium-high heat and add oil.

2. Peel and chop garlic and onion.

3. Put garlic, onion, and sausage in the pot and stir.

4. Cook for few minutes until browned.

5. Pour in chicken stock; add radishes and spinach, stir.

6. Bring mixture to simmer and add cream, bacon, black pepper, salt, and red pepper flakes, stir well.

7. Simmer for 20 minutes.

8. Serve hot.

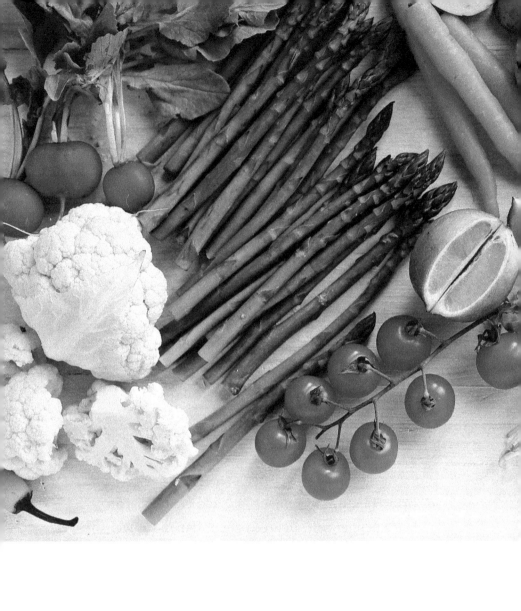

CHAPTER 11

VEGETABLES

CABBAGE HASH BROWNS

PREPARATION
10 MINS

COOKING
12 MINS

SERVINGS
2

INGREDIENTS

- Ingredients
- 1 ½ cup shredded cabbage
- 2 slices of bacon
- 1/2 tsp garlic powder
- 1 egg

- Seasoning:
- 1 tbsp coconut oil
- ½ tsp salt
- 1/8 tsp ground black pepper

NUTRIRION

- Calories: 336
- Fats: 29.5 g
- Protein: 16 g

- Net Carbohydrates: 0.9 g
- Fiber: 0.8 g

DIRECTIONS

1. Crack the egg in a bowl, add garlic powder, black pepper, and salt, whisk well, then add cabbage, toss until well mixed and shape the mixture into four patties.

2. Take a large skillet pan, place it over medium heat, add oil and when hot, add patties in it and cook for 3 minutes per side until golden brown.

3. Transfer hash browns to a plate, then add bacon into the pan and cook for 5 minutes until crispy.

4. Serve hash browns with bacon.

CAULIFLOWER HASH BROWNS

PREPARATION
10 MINS

COOKING
18 MINS

SERVINGS
2

INGREDIENTS

- ¾ cup grated cauliflower t
- 2 slices of bacon
- 1/2 tsp garlic powder
- 1 large egg white

- Seasoning:
- 1 tbsp coconut oil
- ½ tsp salt
- 1/8 tsp ground black pepper

NUTRIRION

- Calories: 347.8
- Fats: 31 g
- Protein: 15.6 g

- Net Carbohydrates: 1.2 g
- Fiber: 0.5 g

DIRECTIONS

1. Place grated cauliflower in a heatproof bowl, cover with plastic wrap, poke some holes in it with a fork and then microwave for 3 minutes until tender.

2. Let steamed cauliflower cool for 10 minutes, then wrap in a cheesecloth and squeeze well to drain moisture as much as possible.

3. Crack the egg in a bowl, add garlic powder, black pepper, and salt, whisk well, then add cauliflower and toss until well mixed and sticky mixture comes together.

4. Take a large skillet pan, place it over medium heat, add oil and when hot, drop cauliflower mixture on it, press lightly to form hash brown patties, and cook for 3 to 4 minutes per side until browned.

5. Transfer hash browns to a plate, then add bacon into the pan and cook for 5 minutes until crispy.

6. Serve hash browns with bacon.

Asparagus, With Bacon and Eggs

PREPARATION
5 MINS

COOKING
12 MINS

SERVINGS
2

INGREDIENTS

- 4 oz asparagus

- 2 slices of bacon, diced

- 1 egg

- Seasoning:

- ¼ tsp salt

- 1/8 tsp ground black pepper

NUTRIRION

- Calories: 179

- Fats: 15.3 g

- Protein: 9 g

- Net Carbohydrates: 0.7 g

- Fiber: 0.6 g

DIRECTIONS

1. Take a skillet pan, place it over medium heat, add bacon, and cook for 4 minutes until crispy.

2. Transfer cooked bacon to a plate, then add asparagus into the pan and cook for 5 minutes until tender-crisp.

3. Crack the egg over the cooked asparagus, season with salt and black pepper, then switch heat to medium-low level and cook for 2 minutes until the egg white has set.

4. Chop the cooked bacon slices, sprinkle over egg and asparagus and serve.

BELL PEPPER EGGS

PREPARATION
10 MINS

COOKING
4 MINS

SERVINGS
2

INGREDIENTS

- 1 green bell pepper

- 2 eggs

- Seasoning:

- 1 tsp coconut oil

- ¼ tsp salt

- ¼ tsp ground black pepper

NUTRIRION

- Calories: 110.5

- Fats: 8 g

- Protein: 7.2 g

- Net Carbohydrates: 1.7 g

- Fiber: 1.1 g

DIRECTIONS

1. Prepare pepper rings, and for this, cut out two slices from the pepper, about ¼-inch, and reserve remaining bell pepper for later use.

2. Take a skillet pan, place it over medium heat, grease it with oil, place pepper rings in it, and then crack an egg into each ring.

3. Season eggs with salt and black pepper, cook for 4 minutes, or until eggs have cooked to the desired level.

4. Transfer eggs to a plate and serve.

OMELET-STUFFED PEPPERS

PREPARATION
5 MINS

COOKING
20 MINS

SERVINGS
2

INGREDIENTS

- 1 large green bell pepper, halved, cored

- 2 eggs

- 2 slices of bacon, chopped, cooked

- 2 tbsp grated parmesan cheese

- Seasoning:

- 1/3 tsp salt

- ¼ tsp ground black pepper

NUTRIRION

- Calories: 428

- Fats: 35.2 g

- Protein: 23.5 g

- Net Carbohydrates: 2.8 g

- Fiber: 1.5

DIRECTIONS

1. Directions:

2. Turn on the oven, then set it to 400 degrees F, and let preheat.

3. Then take a baking dish, pour in 1 tbsp water, place bell pepper halved in it, cut-side up, and bake for 5 minutes.

4. Meanwhile, crack eggs in a bowl, add chopped bacon and cheese, season with salt and black pepper, and whisk until combined.

5. After 5 minutes of baking time, remove baking dish from the oven, evenly fill the peppers with egg mixture and continue baking for 15 to 20 minutes until eggs have set.

6. Serve.

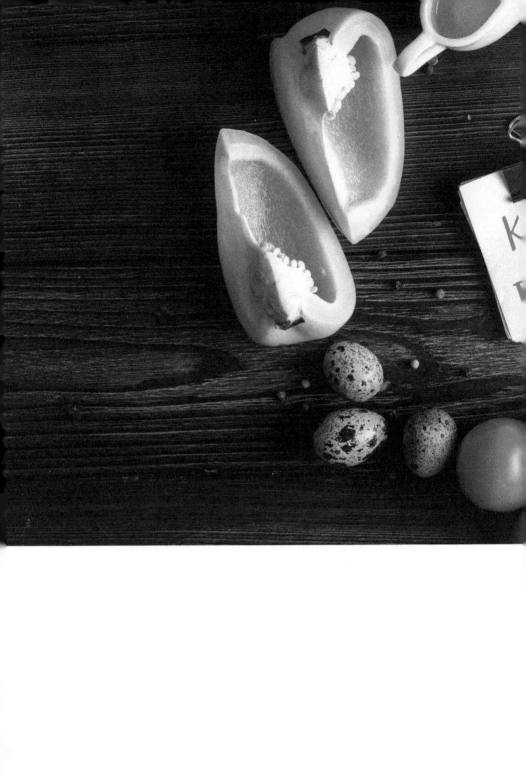

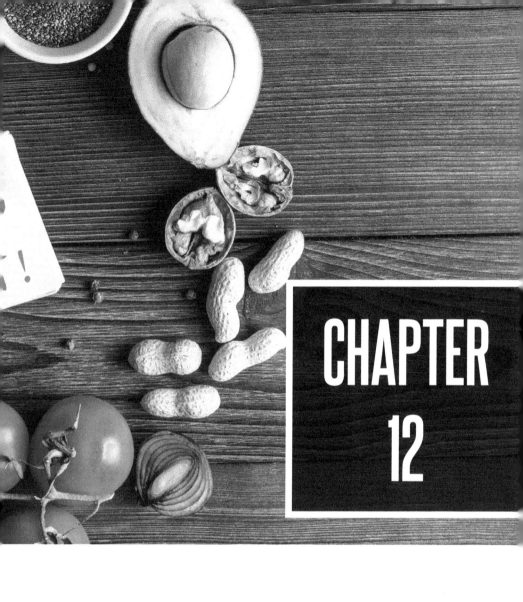

CHAPTER 12

CONCLUSION

Conclusion

The ketogenic diet is one that has many important aspects and information that you need to know as someone who wants to try this diet. It is important to remember the warning that we have given you at the beginning of the book that this is not a diet that is safe and that doctors don't recommend to try it, and if you are going to attempt it remember that you shouldn't do so for longer than six months and even then never without the constant supervision of a doctor or at the very least a doctor knowing that you're doing this and that you're following their guidelines and words to the letter so they can make sure you are safe.

The ketogenic diet is a diet that believes that by minimizing your carbs while maximizing the good fat in your system and making sure that you're getting the protein you need, you will be happier and healthier. In this guidebook, we give you the information to know what this diet is all about, as well as describing the different types and areas that this diet will offer. Most people assume that there is only one way to do this and while there is one thing that the additional options share, there are actually four different options you can choose from. Each one has its unique benefits, and you should know about each type to learn what would be best for your body, which is why we have described them in the book for you to have the best information possible when you begin this diet for yourself.

Another big thing about this diet is that many people don't understand the importance of exercise with this diet. The best way to become healthier is to do three things for yourself. Get the right amount of sleep, eat healthily, and make sure that you get the proper amount of exercise as well for your body to work at an optimum level. The exercises, such as the ones that we explained, are the best to go with your diet to make sure that you are getting the most out of it.

For women who are on the go and have a busy lifestyle, we have provided recipes for a thirty-day meal plan so that you can make food quickly and have a great meal for your lifestyle. They also have enough servings for you to have leftovers so that you don't have to worry about preparing more food in the morning. Instead, you can simply pack it up and take it with you wherever you go. This works out so much easier for so many people because they don't have to cook in the morning, and it saves a busy person a lot of time.

With all of this information at your fingertips, you will be able to enjoy this diet and use it to your advantage. Another benefit that we offer? We explain routines that you can do for yourself to make this diet last longer for you and to benefit your body better as a result. Routines are very important and can be a big help to your body but also your spirit and your mind. Good luck with your keto journey!

CPSIA information can be obtained
at www.ICGtesting.com
Printed in the USA
BVHW091053220221
600778BV00006B/368

9 781801 576420